SERIAL KILLERS
IN HEALTHCARE

SERIAL KILLERS IN HEALTHCARE

Paula Lampe

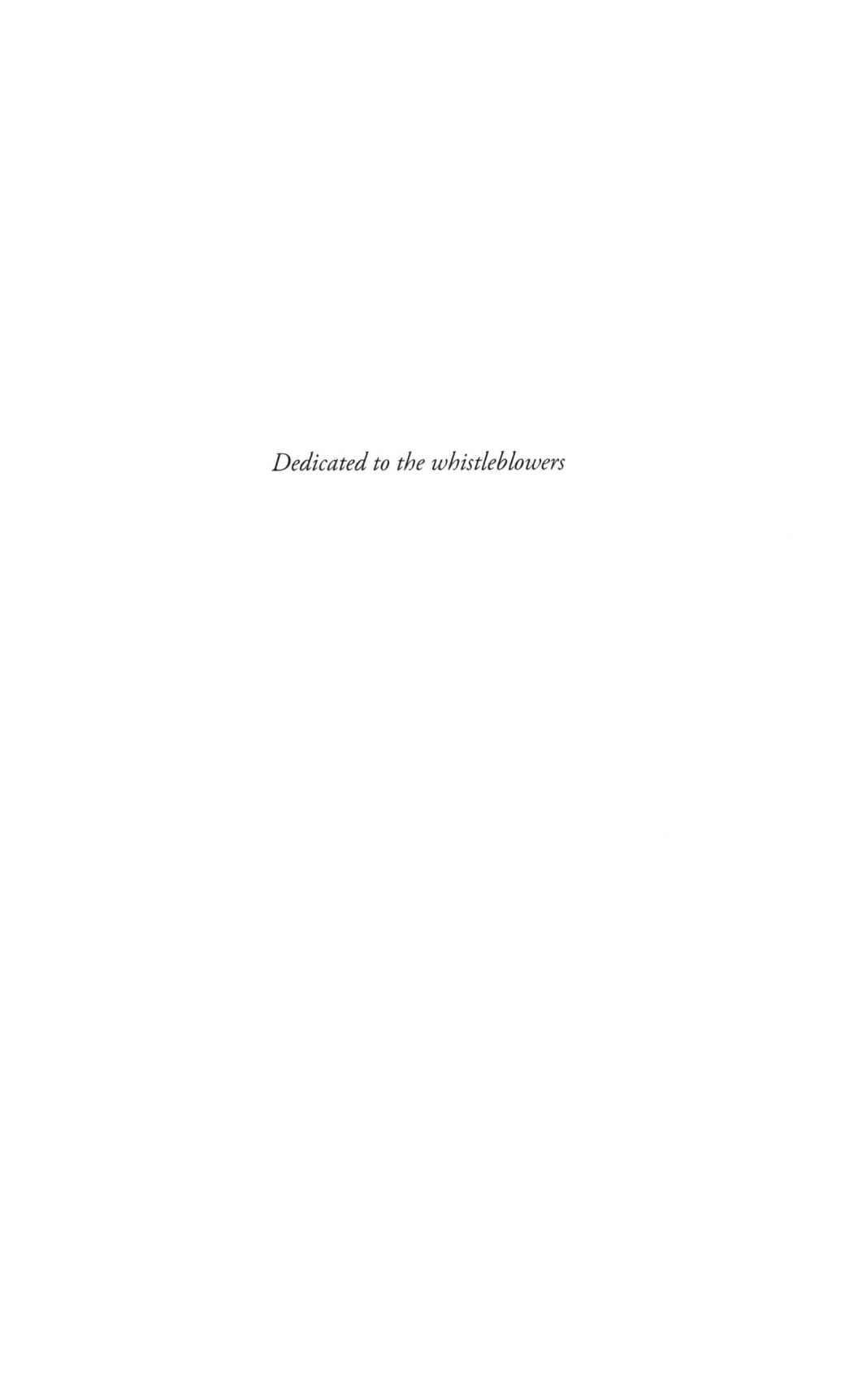

Dedicated to the whistleblowers

CONTENTS

Introduction

Reality often can be stranger than fiction, and that is precisely the case in this book. Serial killers in healthcare are typically affable individuals, beloved by their patients. Take the case of Dr. Shipman, in the final chapter, he was by far the most adored general practitioner in his area. In fact, some of his later victims went to great lengths to secure a spot at the top of his waiting list. When he was finally apprehended, his patients revolted. No one could lay a finger on 'their Fred'. Little did they know that 'Fred' had been administering lethal doses of morphine to his non-terminal patients for a staggering twenty-five years. It was only after a lengthy investigation and an exhaustive trial that he was convicted of fifteen murders and suspected of 225 more. It was then that the horrifying truth began to sink in.

But hang on a moment! A doctor murdering his patients? Aren't these so-called healthcare murders mere fantasy? After all, in the Netherlands, a nurse who had been imprisoned for years for murder was ultimately acquitted of the charges because, during the reopening of the case, there was nothing left of the so-called 'evidence' in legal terms. Despite the seemingly compelling evidence presented during her 2002 trial and the subsequent 2004 appeal, when all was said and done, her guilt dissolved, as it should, if it no longer legally stands.

Does this mean however, that healthcare serial killers are non-existent? Such doubt is understandable, and to provide a conclusive response, we must thoroughly examine this phenomenon on a global level. This investigation has been carried out, and research data don't lie.

As early as 1883, Danish childcare provider Dagmar Johanne Amalie Overbye took the lives of between nine and twenty-five children. It wasn't until a century later, in 1988, that (at present) professor emerita of nursing and criminal justice & criminalistics Beatrice Yorker initially raised the issue. She noticed a connection between nurses who killed their patients and the Munchausen by Proxy syndrome (where a mother harms her child in order to gain attention herself), initially termed Factitious Disorder by Proxy (FDP), which roughly translates to 'resembling Munchausen by Proxy syndrome.' English pediatric nurse Beverley Allitt from Chapter 11 and American nurse Genene Jones from Chapter 12 were even diagnosed with this syndrome. Beverley received thirteen life sentences for the murder of four children and the attempted murder of eight. Genene received a life sentence plus sixty years for one murder, one attempted murder, and an additional 27 suspected victims.

Forensic toxicologist Robert Forrest wrote his doctoral thesis on healthcare serial killers in 1992: *Investigation of Health Care Workers who Systematically Harm their Patients* (1992). He introduced not one but two new terms: 'Carer Associated Serial Killing (CASK)' and 'Carer Associated Serial Homicide (CASH)'.

In 1998, Karl Heinz Beine followed with his book *Sehen, Hören, Schweigen. Patiententötungen und Aktive Sterbehilfe* (Seeing, Hearing and Keeping Quiet. Patient Killing and Active Euthanasia). Beine had previously worked as a psychiatrist on the same ward where the perpetrator Wolfgang Lange, from Chapter 14, later murdered nine patients. Beine conducted research into 28 similar cases. Alongside the Dutch term I introduced, 'Seriemoordenaars in de gezondheidszorg (SMGZ),' (Serial Killers in Healthcare) two other designations have been used: 'Caregiver Associated Epidemics (CAE)' and 'Health Care Serial Murder (HCSM)', all abbreviations used to refer to serial killings committed by healthcare personnel.

Beatrice Yorker and her co-authors, including myself, then conducted research that resulted in the 2006 publication *Serial Murder by Healthcare Professionals* in the prestigious *American Journal of Forensic Science*. Yorker continues tirelessly to raise awareness of the issue. The most recent term she introduced is 'Nosocomial Homicide', meaning 'homicide during medical treatment.' As a consequence of these publications, continuous global research is underway with the aim of bringing healthcare serial killers to justice.

The findings of *Serial Murder by Healthcare Professionals* can be summarized as follows: Healthcare serial killers have been found in many countries. In the thirty years leading up to this research, 54 perpetrators were convicted of multiple murders or attempted murders. Which makes the likelihood of falling victim to a healthcare serial killer roughly equivalent to the chance of being struck by lightning. And although it is rare to meet one's end in such a manner, we do take precautions against lightning strikes. Plus it's worth noting that the number of discovered murderers is on the rise, partly due to research. Besides a few physicians, the vast majority of perpetrators occur in the nursing and caregiving professions, which is not surprising given that the number of nursing, caregiving, and paramedical personnel exceeds that of physicians. Noteworthy is however, the overrepresentation of men. Although they are a minority in this sector, research found that forty-four percent of the perpetrators were male. Ninety-nine percent of the convicted individuals were of Caucasian descent. The majority of victims occurred in hospitals during the evening or night shifts, when working alone is more prevalent. Victims under one year of age or over seventy were the most susceptible, which can be attributed to their reduced resilience.

The 54 perpetrators were convicted of a total of 328 murders and 130 cases of manslaughter or attempted murder. However, to reach a verdict, guilt must be proven beyond reasonable doubt. Since deaths in healthcare institutions are considered normal, where contact between the perpetrator and victim is more the rule than the exception, murder could not always be proven. Meaning, involvement of defendants in the suspicious deaths of 2,113 patients could not be supported by legitimate evidence. Various convicted perpetrators used more than one method to commit murder. The most common method was administering an overdose of medications, alongside strangulation, drowning, disabling equipment, and poisoning.

The question that has been troubling everyone is why healthcare professionals would intentionally prematurely terminate the lives of their patients. Suspects motives (if they admit that is) do not always correspond with what professionals believe motivated them. Many of the accused argue that they acted out of compassion, viewing their actions as a form of euthanasia with unintended mistakes. At times, suspects cite being overburden, claiming they simply wanted to 'empty beds'.

Since 2001, the Netherlands has been a pioneer in the realm of euthanasia, which is no longer a criminal offense. As long as it adheres within legal boundaries; meaning, the procedure solely being reserved for medical doctors. However, as we know, most perpetrators come from the caregiving or nursing sector.

Moreover, in most examined cases, there was no mention of unbearable suffering. In fact, most victims weren't even terminally ill. Murder occurring covertly, without deliberating with the victim's family or with colleagues. Compassion couldn't be attributed to the patient's unbearable suffering. Victims were admitted for minor procedures, were on the mend, or arbitrarily killed without any knowledge of the victim nor their prognosis. Experts however are more inclined believing perpetrators could not bear the suffering of others themselves. Additionally, a small number of convicted individuals had a history of brain damage.

Noticeably were the striking similarities in perpetrators profiles. Most had a significantly diminished sense of self-worth, with 'helping' being a way to validate their existence, as I described in my book: *Het Moeder Teresasyndroom* (The Mother Teresa Syndrome, 2002). Quite a few seemed to be seeking 'drama', administering an overdose, in order playing the hero during resuscitation. This need for craving the spotlight aligning with the frequently observed narcissistic personality.

Culprits were socially emotionally withdrawn individuals who led solitary lives, maintaining an isolated position within the department. Several had criminal records. Prior to the unmasking of the suspected perpetrator, rumors circulated while whistleblowers were almost invariably ignored. Raising concern that the number of cases might, in essence, even be greater.

Successively, 23 European and American cases are described in this book. By no means implying that healthcare serial killers do not exist in Asia, the Middle East, South America, and Africa.

All perpetrators were convicted, either because they confessed or were seen by an eyewitness, or because the corroborating evidence was overwhelming and compelling. For instance, unexplained deaths occurred not only at one workplace but across multiple locations where they worked, and excessive deaths ceasing after their departure. Furthermore, an overdose of medications was confirmed by the pathologist in the deceased.

While all facts are accurately portrayed, some atmosphere has been added for readability. The fact that the last case described in this book was discovered in 2007 unfortunately doesn't mean that such murders have ceased to occur. Since then, individuals for instance like the American nurse Kimberly Saenz (2008), the Finnish nurses Katariina Pantila Loennqvist (2009) and Aino Nykopp-Koski (2010), the Spanish aide Joan Vila (2010), the Australian nurse Roger Kingsley (2011), the Canadian nurse Elizabeth Mae Wettlaufer (2016) and not to forget the English neonatal nurse Lucy Letby (2017) and more, have been sentenced to lengthy, sometimes lifelong imprisonment. Others are still awaiting trial.

With this book, I hope to clarify why serial murders can occur worldwide in locations, by no one expected, committed by personnel who are beyond suspicion, in a manner that everyone deems utterly impossible. So that when an unexpectedly high number of patients die in the presence of the same caregiver, without hesitation law enforcement will be contacted.

Paula Lampe, Amsterdam, 2024
schrijfenblijf@gmail.com

1.

Broken trust

Frans H., The Netherlands, 1972

Double Arrest

In the serene stretches of Limburg, a province cradled in the southern embrace of The Netherlands, the police commissioner found himself thrust into a chilling conundrum. It began with a call that pierced the tranquility of his office, a call that whispered of potential murderer lurking within the shadows of the Luckerheide Clinic in Kerkrade. At first, skepticism danced in the commissioner's mind like a devil's waltz. It seemed too macabre, too surreal to be anything but a cruel jest. Yet, as the officer's voice cracked with urgency, the commissioner's disbelief thawed, replaced by a steely resolve. He knew he couldn't afford the luxury of doubt. With a grim determination etched upon his features, he raced through the winding roads, his thoughts entangled in the web of impending dread.

Upon reaching the scene, he wasted no time. Gathering a cadre of investigators, their grim expressions mirrored the weight of the darkness that loomed ahead. This was no ordinary case, and the commissioner understood the stakes all too well. With a sense of urgency that bordered on desperation, he made a crucial decision, summoning the aid of the national investigative police.

The die was cast; the stage was set for the unraveling of a mystery that had long haunted the corridors of the clinic. November's chill hung heavy in the air, casting an eerie pall over the tranquil landscape of Limburg. Like specters in a shadow play, the investigators descended upon the Nightingale ward, their every step a testament to the relentless pursuit of truth.

Their quarry was a colossus of a man, the head nurse, his imposing frame belying the darkness that lurks within. In his possession, a wallet bulging with 719 guilders in total. A sum dismissed as mere pocket change, until the investigators revealed a sinister truth. Beneath the facade of innocence lay a thief, pilfering clothing allowances meant for the most vulnerable souls under his care.

Frans was a man of fierce defiance. When confronted with accusations, his response was a torrent of denial, a vehement protestation that he was a victim of a sinister plot. He distanced himself from the grim tally of deaths haunting his domain, his fury erupting like molten lava. Through the corridors, his voice thundered, each scream a testament to his unraveling composure until, at last, he surrendered to the overwhelming torrent of emotions, tears staining his cheeks as the tempest within him raged unchecked.

Yet, with the dawn of a new day, a metamorphosis seized him. The once tempestuous outbursts gave way to a stoic silence. He became a master of evasion, deflecting every inquiry with practiced finesse, his responses veiled in layers of ambiguity. 'What do you mean?' he would counter. 'Do you even comprehend the intricacies of medicine?' or 'I like to talk to my mother.' His demeanor underwent a profound transformation, a shift so palpable that even his attorney bore witness to the dramatic change.

Then came the moment of reckoning. With a furtive glance at his counselor, balancing on the edge of his chair, with tears streaming down his cheeks, Frans confessed. In the rustic cadence of the Limburg dialect, he admitted to the unspeakable, administering fatal doses of insulin or valium to fifteen patients.

The narrative took a surreal turn, as if the very essence of human depravity had been laid bare in that chilling confession. A hush fell over the room, broken only by the sound of Frans's ragged breathing. Once again, he sought the advice of his lawyer. But he shook his head disapprovingly and with an air of arrogance Frans withdrew his confession and remarked disdainfully in impeccable Standard Dutch: 'You can't even kill a patient with insulin.'

As the interrogation sessions continued, a new facet of Frans emerged, a facet common among serial killers in the healthcare profession. Gone was the disheveled figure of earlier questioning; now, he sat poised and collected, exuding an aura of confidence that seemed to defy the gravity of his situation. With a demeanor reminiscent of a physician conducting a routine examination, he calmly acknowledged his transgressions. Admitting to the unlawful administration of medications, he spoke with a sense of liberation, as if unburdening his soul of long-held secrets. His justification? A misguided attempt to alleviate suffering and lighten the workload of his colleagues, burdened by the relentless demands of their profession. Little did the detectives realize then the depths of Frans's compulsions, his mind consumed by a relentless obsession with cleanliness, driving him to the brink of psychological collapse during his months of pretrial detention.

The investigative team found themselves ensnared in a web of deception and horror as they combed through Frans's domain. Each hidden treasure unearthed whispered of betrayal and deceit, painting a chilling portrait of the man behind the nurse's uniform. With each discovery, the list of charges against him grew: fourteen counts of murder intertwined with theft, his crimes extending far beyond the boundaries of mere mortality. Among the macabre finds was a stolen necklace, carefully packaged and placed beneath a glittering Christmas tree, a perverse gift for his unsuspecting wife.

Yet, even as the judge delivered the verdict, a pall of uncertainty lingered over the countless death certificates signed by Frans. In 112 cases, doubt cast a shadow over the supposed natural causes of death, leaving a haunting question mark hanging over the proceedings.

For the police commissioner, once dismissive of what seemed an absurd prank, the reality had become chillingly clear. This was no joke; it was the unraveling of one of the most extensive murder investigations in Dutch history, a tale that would haunt the nation for years to come.

Amidst the labyrinthine darkness of Frans's crimes, another startling revelation emerged. Delving into the enigmatic world of the Nightingale ward, investigators turned their gaze to Frans's mother. A seemingly innocuous conversation took a sinister turn as she disclosed the troubling symptoms afflicting her second husband, symptoms hinting at poisoning. While suspicion initially fell upon Frans, careful scrutiny unveiled a shocking truth: the perpetrator was none other than his own mother. In a twist that sent shockwaves through the investigation, she would ultimately stand convicted of attempted murder, casting a shadow of doubt even over the bonds of familial trust.

A Model Employee

Frans's journey began amidst the cobbled streets of Kerkrade in 1935, a town steeped in the rich history of Western Europe's mining legacy. Born as the third son in a devout Catholic family, his early years were marked by the challenges of a congenital condition, a cleft lip. Hospitalizations for corrective surgeries fostered a deep bond between Frans and his mother, shaping the foundation of their relationship. With a little sister joining the family fold, Frans's formative years unfolded against the backdrop of familial love and resilience.

After completing his high school, Frans toiled in a factory before heeding the call to serve as a nurse. His training in Sittard set the stage for a career dedicated to healing, but a yearning for spiritual fulfillment led him to the threshold of the Order of Saint Joseph. Clad in the garb of a novice, Frans embarked on a path of devotion, only to realize the mismatch between his aspirations and the rigors of monastic life. Returning to the secular realm, he found solace in the halls of a regional hospital before fate guided him to the Nightingale ward of the Luckerheide clinic.

In July 1972, at the age of 39, his father passed away. Within six months, his mother remarried to a widower whose late wife happened to have been admitted to the Luckerheide clinic before her death. The relationship between Frans and his stepfather soured when the widower recognized a stolen sweater that had belonged to his deceased wife, a gift Frans had accidentally given to his mother.

The year 1974 cast a somber pall over Kerkrade, a town etched with the indelible marks of its mining heritage. Against this backdrop, the Luckerheide clinic stood as a bastion of comfort, a sanctuary where the elderly of Kerkrade could find solace in the twilight of their years. Yet, within the confines of this haven, a curious tale began to weave its threads, centering on Frans, a head nurse with an idiosyncratic obsession, tending to the Virgin Mary statue in the chapel with almost religious zeal and performing uncharacteristic tasks like dusting nightstands and making beds. An unconventional role for a man in his position, to be sure. Approaching his duties with a meticulousness that bordered on the inexplicable, earning him both admiration and curiosity from his peers. As the days turned into weeks, the enigmatic aura surrounding Frans only deepened, casting a veil of intrigue over the Nightingale ward and the man who tended to its inhabitants with unwavering devotion.

Nurse Frans cast a long shadow over the clinic, a figure of authority forged by nineteen years of unwavering dedication to his craft. With a laundry list of titles, works council member, staff association chairman, and training committee member, he wielded influence that stretched far beyond the confines of his ward. To those around him, he exuded an air of invincibility, his confidence unshakable, his position seemingly beyond reproach.

Yet, beneath the facade of professional prowess lurked a chilling undercurrent of suspicion. It began with a casual remark from the head of the nursing department, a jest veiled in the guise of humor but pregnant with ominous implications. 'Patients disappearing through the back door so quickly, we can't admit them fast enough through the front door,' he quipped to Frans, a seemingly innocuous comment that hinted at something far more sinister lurking beneath the surface.

Since assuming his role as head nurse in 1972, the same year his father passed away, a pattern of death had emerged within the Nightingale ward, a pattern as unsettling as it was inexplicable. Patients, regardless of their health status upon admission, seemed to succumb to the embrace of death with alarming swiftness. Even those destined for long-term care were not spared from the grip of this enigma.

In the close-knit community of Kerkrade and its surroundings, whispers of suspicion danced through the air like specters in the night. The elderly, seasoned by the passage of time, understood all too well the fragility of life within the walls of the Luckerheide clinic. While the alarmingly high mortality rate remained largely confined to the Nightingale ward, it did not escape notice that many who entered its doors never emerged again. Even the local physicians, attuned to the ebb and flow of life, raised an eyebrow at the unnaturally short lifespans that seemed to plague the clinic's inhabitants.

Yet, amidst the murmurs and rumors, one unsettling truth remained: the puzzle of the Nightingale ward's mortality rate remained largely unexplored, a shadowy specter lurking just beyond the reach of those who should have known better.

Hamster

In the balmy days of June 1975, a fresh-faced doctor stepped into her new role, but her enthusiasm soon collided with a chilling reality, a reality painted with the brushstrokes of death. Within days of her arrival, she found herself ensnared in a web of eerie occurrences, as an unsettling pattern emerged: an unnaturally high number of patients meeting their demise within the Nightingale ward's confines.

It was a singular event that served as the catalyst for her reckoning, a sudden death that sent shockwaves reverberating through the corridors, leaving an indelible mark upon her psyche. Innocent inquiries unveiled cryptic whispers that hung heavy in the air, haunting reminders of a truth too sinister to ignore. 'Where nurse Frans is, more patients die', the ominous refrain echoed, igniting a firestorm of suspicion within the doctor's soul.

With steely determination, she summoned each member of the staff to her office, coaxing forth their hidden truths with gentle persuasion. Slowly, hesitations gave way to confessions, and a torrent of unsettling tales spilled forth. The doctor listened with bated breath as caregivers unburdened themselves, revealing the grim reality of a mortality rate spiraling out of control. Their cries for change had fallen on deaf ears, their pleas for intervention met with callous indifference.

Embedded within the accounts of Frans's coworkers lay chilling details, each revelation more disturbing than the last. The mysterious disappearance of insulin, borrowed under dubious circumstances, had earned Frans the sinister moniker of 'Hamster.' As suspicion mounted, a courageous colleague dared to venture into the heart of darkness, the refrigerator on the Nightingale ward. What he discovered, or rather, what he did not find, left him reeling in disbelief. The insulin supply, depleted to near exhaustion, painted a damning portrait of deception and betrayal. Yet, when he raised the alarm, the response was not one of urgency but of dismissive incredulity. That this will not be the last case where whistleblowers are not taken seriously will become clear to the reader in the course of this book. Whispers of a thief lurking in the shadows cast a pall of fear over the clinic, where patients' belongings vanished without a trace, swallowed by the voracious maw of darkness.

But the darkness lurking within the walls of the clinic was far from complete. A caregiver, with trembling hands and a heart heavy with dread, bore witness to Frans's sinister machinations. In the final moments before a patient's untimely demise, Frans administered a dubious injection, his actions shrouded in the cloak of deception. And as life ebbed away, he surreptitiously tampered with the oxygen supply, sealing the victim's fate with a chilling finality.

Frans's reign of terror extended beyond the realm of life and death. Allegedly decreeing that all deaths be meticulously recorded in a notebook, he imposed his will upon the ward with an iron fist, silencing dissenting voices with a cold indifference. His directives stood in stark contrast to the opinions of his peers, a testament to his unchecked authority and unyielding grip on power.

But it was the whispers in the night that sent shivers down the spine of the clinic's inhabitants. From the comfort of his home, Frans would call with eerie precision, inquiring about the condition of those teetering on the brink of death or newly discovered lifeless in their beds. His calls, laden with a sinister intent, echoed through the halls like a harbinger of doom.

As the newly arrived physician stepped into the fray, she wasted no time in taking command. With a resolve as unyielding as the steel of her scalpel, she confronted the clinic's administration with a dire warning of imminent action. Her words, dripping with ominous portent, left them with no choice but to heed her call.

In a whirlwind of authority, police officers and Health Inspectorate officials descended upon the clinic, their presence a beacon of hope amidst the encroaching darkness. With each passing moment, the intricate web of enigma and malevolence began to unravel, exposing the chilling secrets hidden within the hallowed halls of the Nightingale ward.

Women's Clothing

The staff, comprised of both family members of patients and grieving relatives, found themselves thrust into a maelstrom of disbelief and uncertainty. The unthinkable notion that a murderer could be lurking within the hallowed halls of the Luckerheide Clinic sent shockwaves rippling through their ranks. And when the beloved head nurse of the Nightingale ward was led away in handcuffs, the chaos reached a fever pitch.

It was a scenario beyond comprehension: a dedicated caregiver accused of the most heinous of crimes. Surely, the police must be mistaken. Perhaps nurse Frans, in his misguided attempt to alleviate suffering, had merely hastened the inevitable for those trapped in the throes of unbearable pain. Such thoughts, though irrational, offered a modicum of solace amidst the tumult.

As concerned parties rallied to nurse Frans's defense, the outpouring of support served as a testament to the profound disbelief that often accompanies the arrest of a suspected serial killer in the healthcare sector. Deliberately causing the deaths of patients was deemed unfathomable, and yet, the subsequent show of solidarity seemed almost surreal in hindsight.

Distraught family members grappled with a newfound fear, questioning whether their loved ones were truly safe within the confines of the facility. Amidst the uncertainty, the staff of the Nightingale ward found themselves enveloped in a blanket of relief, their faith in their colleague's innocence unwavering.

But as the legal machinery churned forward, bringing with it a litany of charges including fourteen counts of murder, theft, forgery, and embezzlement, a tumultuous legal battle unfolded. Frans H. stood defiant, steadfast in his belief that he had been coerced and manipulated by the authorities. Even within the confines of the courtroom, he refused to yield, frequently interrupting proceedings with a brazen disregard for decorum.

Judges and prosecutors, renowned for their stoicism, found themselves tested by the eccentric behavior of the defendant. Stern reprimands echoed through the courtroom, warning Frans of the consequences should he persist in disrupting the proceedings. Yet, amidst the chaos and uncertainty, one truth remained immutable, the chilling specter of death that had cast its shadow over the Nightingale ward would not be easily vanquished.

As the prosecutor laid bare the details of the case, a chilling portrait of deceit and manipulation emerged. Within the confines of Frans's residence, stolen women's clothing lay hidden, a macabre collection amassed under the guise of innocence. Authorized to make purchases on behalf of patients, Frans had exploited his position of trust, withholding purchased women's suits in his wife's size with a cunning that defied detection. Nearly fifty items of clothing, pilfered from the vulnerable under his care, bore silent witness to his treachery. And yet, no one had ever suspected a thing.

But Frans's ingenuity knew no bounds. Not content with mere theft, he had devised a scheme to profit from his ill-gotten gains, selling some of the stolen garments at a modest price to his unsuspecting relatives. To further cement his deception, he had submitted claims to social services for a higher amount than the clothing had cost him, lining his pockets with the proceeds of his crimes.

In his defense, Frans sought to deflect blame, insinuating that he was not the sole perpetrator of such activities within the clinic's walls. Yet, as the evidence unfolded, his assertions crumbled under the weight of scrutiny.

A meticulous examination of the timeline revealed a damning pattern. A quarter of patients admitted to the Nightingale ward met their demise on the first day, with thirty percent passing away by the second. Within a week of admission, half had succumbed to the embrace of death, a statistic that defied explanation. In contrast, on all other wards combined, the mortality rate remained staggeringly low.

Further analysis unearthed additional anomalies. Among non-diabetic patients on the Nightingale ward, a disproportionate number fell victim to diabetic coma, an affliction unheard of among their counterparts on other wards. And in a twist of fate, unexplained deaths on alternate wards coincided with Frans's temporary assignment, raising suspicions of foul play.

In essence, between 1972 and 1975, a staggering 259 patients met their demise under suspicious circumstances, primarily on the Nightingale ward, an alarming statistic that bore the unmistakable imprint of Frans's presence. As the evidence mounted, the facade of innocence crumbled, leaving behind a trail of devastation and despair in its wake.

Pattern

Let's delve into the chilling mechanics of Frans's crimes, a dark saga fraught with manipulation and malice. But first, a glimpse into the lives of his victims, frail individuals teetering on the brink of mortality. Aged between 68 and 93, they were ensnared by a web of dependency, their bodies ravaged by illness and their minds clouded by the fog of dementia. For many, the scars of a lifetime of toil in the mines lingered, their lungs poisoned by the insidious grip of silicosis, a grim reminder of their labor in the depths of the earth.

Initially targeting male victims, Frans's sinister agenda soon expanded to encompass women as well, leaving no soul untouched by his malevolent hand. Half of his confessed murders were executed with a lethal overdose of insulin, while the remainder succumbed to the venomous embrace of Valium. Yet, the exact circumstances surrounding the suspected number of deaths, ranging from 112 to 259, remain shrouded in mystery, a testament to the calculated cunning of a man consumed by darkness.

Despite the defense's assertions of emotional strain, Frans's actions betray a chilling precision. His injections, administered with a steady hand and unwavering resolve, left little room for doubt. Witness testimony revealed a sinister pattern: injections strategically timed during the bustle of feeding time or even in the presence of visitors, the facade of innocence maintained until the final, fatal dose was delivered.

Upon the request of the Prosecution, pharmacy orders were meticulously examined. The head nurse of the Nightingale ward ordered 88 more vials of insulin than necessary for the patient population during the suspected period. Within three days after his vacation, Nurse Frans managed to gather a quantity of insulin that the inspector couldn't find after his arrest. Just before the weekend, he allegedly predicted, 'Let's bet who will have died by Monday...'

Foul-Mouthing

In the quiet moments of reflection, family members grappled with the unthinkable, could the very man entrusted with their loved one's care be harboring a deadly secret? While suspicions simmered beneath the surface, shrouded in the cloak of disbelief, subtle hints of Frans's malevolence began to emerge.

Inappropriate remarks, uttered with a chilling nonchalance, lingered in the air like a harbinger of doom. To one family, facing the grim reality of a loved one admitted in critical condition, Frans's words cut like a knife: 'More dead than alive', he declared, a callous disregard for the fragility of life. And as ambulance personnel ushered another soul into the ward's embrace, Frans's muttered words betrayed a sinister intent: 'Feeble soul', he sneered, his tone dripping with contempt.

But it was the precision of his words that sent shivers down the spine of a concerned daughter, her mother's life hanging in the balance. 'Three-quarters of an hour,' Frans declared with a chilling certainty, his timing eerily precise. And when asked about the need for a shot, his answer: 'liver shot' sounded hollow, a blatant lie cloaked in deceit.

Yet, it was the callousness of his remarks that pierced the veil of innocence, leaving a trail of devastation in his wake. To the daughter sitting beside her severely demented mother's bed, he had drunkenly exclaimed: 'If it were up to me, we'd let her go to sleep'. A 75-year-old patient, who was admitted by her children as a cheerful grandma, lay dead in bed within twelve hours.

In the intricate dance of justice, convicting serial killers in healthcare proves a formidable challenge, for the lines between caregiver and perpetrator blur in a realm where trust and betrayal intertwine. Unlike traditional criminal cases, establishing guilt hinges not on direct evidence but on a meticulous unraveling of statistical anomalies, a task fraught with complexity and nuance.

Enter the statistician, a silent sentinel of truth in the courtroom, whose expertise lies in deciphering the cryptic patterns hidden within the web of deceit. Armed with duty rosters and timelines of suspicious deaths, they meticulously trace the footprints of the perpetrator, seeking the elusive thread that binds them to their crimes. In Frans's case, the statistician's testimony served as a beacon of clarity amidst the fog of uncertainty, revealing a damning truth.

Through the lens of statistical analysis, the sinister nature of Frans's deeds emerged with chilling clarity. A staggering 82 percent of disputed deaths occurred within his 'responsibility time,' a damning testament to his presence at the scene of the crimes. But it was the broader context that painted the most damning picture, the disproportionate number of deaths on the Nightingale ward, a statistic that defied rational explanation.

Indeed, the statistician's findings left little room for doubt. The odds of 11.7 percent of non-diabetic patients succumbing to diabetic coma on the Nightingale ward, compared to a mere 0.6 percent on all other wards combined, were a statistical anomaly too glaring to ignore. And as the shadows of suspicion loomed large, the statistician's testimony served as a beacon of truth, illuminating the darkness that had shrouded the Nightingale ward for far too long.

The statistician's findings further supported the fact that after the arrest of nurse Frans, no patient in the clinic died within a week of admission until the trial, despite there being 68 admissions.

Mentally Diminished

In the hallowed halls of justice, where truth and deception collide, experts from the psychiatric observation clinic stepped into the spotlight, shedding light on the twisted psyche of the accused. Rooted in Freudian theory, their diagnosis painted a chilling portrait of a man consumed by dark desires and primal urges.

At the core of their analysis lay the concept of an abnormally strong oedipal attachment, a tangled web of longing and resentment, where the lines between son and mother blur into obscurity, viewing the father as a rival.

But it was the stark contradiction between the suspect's profession and his personality that raised the most alarming red flags. Egocentric, dishonest, devoid of empathy, the traits of a man driven by a hunger for power and validation. His low level of intelligence is even less compatible with his role as a head nurse.

His compulsive need for cleanliness points to a character neurosis with compulsive actions, driven by underlying fear. Anything that irritates him must be cleaned up, including troublesome patients who disrupt his routine. Although he commits murder out of self-interest, the final conclusion is that the suspect is only partially responsible for his actions due to his intellectual limitations.

But as the prosecution delivered its damning closing statement, the gravity of the suspect's crimes hung heavy in the air. The trust of society shattered, the integrity of nursing staff called into question, their words echoed with a sense of urgency and indignation. For the loved ones left behind, grief mingled with anger, the specter of uncertainty looming large.

In the face of such atrocities, justice demanded retribution, a punishment befitting the severity of the crimes committed. And as the courtroom fell silent, the weight of their words reverberated, a plea for a life sentence, a beacon of justice in a world darkened by betrayal and despair.

In the labyrinthine corridors of the courtroom, where truth and deceit clash in a battle for justice, the defense emerged with a defiant stance, challenging the very foundation upon which the prosecution's case rested. Casting a shadow of doubt over the proceedings, they painted a damning portrait of a clinic plagued by negligence and a system riddled with flaws.

According to the defense, the blame could not rest solely on their client's shoulders. The nursing home's leadership stood accused of gross negligence, while doctors were lambasted for their dereliction of duty. In a damning indictment of the system, the pharmacist's failure to heed the warning signs of excessive insulin orders was laid bare, a critical oversight that had dire consequences.

But it was the defense's meticulous dismantling of the prosecution's statistical analysis that struck at the heart of their argument. Shift swaps, communication breakdowns, the flaws in the data were laid bare for all to see. And as doubts lingered over the function and effect of insulin, the defense seized upon the uncertainty, demanding answers from the very experts whose testimony had formed the bedrock of the prosecution's case.

With a steely resolve, the defense rallied around their client, demanding an acquittal on grounds of coerced confession, lack of motive, and a tenuous link between insulin administration and patient deaths. And as the courtroom buzzed with speculation, the media descended upon the trial, their watchful eyes casting a spotlight on the proceedings.

But just as the verdict loomed on the horizon, a twist of fate threw the courtroom into disarray, the sudden replacement of the court's president, sparking whispers of doubt and suspicion. In the tumult of uncertainty, two national newspapers dared to question the evidence and the impartiality of the judges, a final twist in a trial fraught with intrigue and uncertainty.

Good Behavior

In the courtroom's solemn chamber, where justice awaited its final reckoning, the verdict fell with a resounding clang, a verdict of murder. Nurse Frans, with his knowledge of insulin's deadly potential, stood accused of wielding a weapon of silent destruction, his actions betraying the very oath he had sworn to uphold.

The prosecution painted a chilling picture of calculated malice, highlighting Frans's deliberate injection of insulin into the unsuspecting bodies of his victims. Each fatal dose, administered with cold precision, bore the mark of a man consumed by darkness, a man who knew all too well the lethal consequences of his actions.

Yet, amidst the damning evidence and the weight of the law, there lingered a haunting specter of complicity, a system marred by incompetence and neglect. While the clinic's shortcomings offered a glimmer of leniency, they paled in comparison to the heinous acts committed by the perpetrator.

Frans H., once a towering figure of authority, now faced the cold embrace of justice, a sentence of thirteen years behind bars, accompanied by twenty-three years of professional disqualification. But even as the gavel fell, sealing his fate, the echoes of his crimes reverberated far beyond the confines of the courtroom. On appeal, the sentence was increased by five years. However, he was released in 1987 after serving twelve years for good behavior and dies in 2006 at the age of 71. As the years passed, and the memory of Nurse Frans faded into the annals of history, his legacy endured, a dark stain on the fabric of society.

The extensive media coverage of this case, however, had a dark side, as Nurse Frans's gruesome activities inspired a colleague in neighboring Belgium.

2.

The nun who ate lobster

Sister Godfrieda, Belgium, 1977

Vocation

In 1933, Cecile emerges into a world of prosperity and privilege. Later shadows loom as one of her sisters succumbs to the relentless grip of bone cancer at twenty-nine, while her other sister, ensnared by the clutches of alcohol addiction, ends up within the walls of a psychiatric institution.

A portrait of innocence, Cecile, with her cherubic countenance, entering school after church, warmly greeted by the sister-nuns. Their tales of divine beckoning become the foundation upon which Cecile builds her devotion. As she ascends through higher education, her piety deepens, and each night she clasps her hands in fervent prayer, seeking fortitude for the journey into the sanctified realms of convent life. On the cusp of her eighteenth birthday, convinced of a divine calling, she boldly declares her intention to join the Holy Apostolines of Saint Joseph in Wetteren, Belgium, a serene enclave near Ghent, nestled in the conservative, Catholic core of the country, where the sisters are the custodians of education and healing.

Post her training as a nurse and midwife, Cecile, a bit shaky, bids a tearful adieu to her parents at the convent gate. As her mother wrestles with her tears, Cecile ambles tentatively towards the weathered, imposing structure.

Her tresses shorn and now christened Sister Godfrieda, the postulant year unfolds, an initiation into convent life with a slightly ajar door. Amidst collective prayers, she engages in mundane tasks: peeling potatoes, baking bread, and ironing habits. Her austere cell, a frigid cocoon, denies her the solace of a restful slumber.

A year elapses, propelling her into the realm of a novice. She can still change her mind or be sent away by Mother Superior. Nonetheless, Sister Godfrieda obediently immerses herself in the scriptures, partakes in the solemn communion, and confesses her innermost thoughts. Two additional years slide by, marking the acceptance of temporary vows. Then, at the age of twenty-four, she stands before God, Holy Mary, and her sisterhood, articulating the eternal vows of poverty, obedience, and celibacy. Draped in her new habit, she bids adieu to her parents once more at the gate, but this time, a resolute stride carries her through the grand entrance, where the mother superior appoints her as the head sister in the geriatric ward of the Saint Joseph hospital, a chapter in Sister Godfrieda's veiled odyssey.

Whispers

In the annals of Wetteren's hospital history, Sister Godfrieda's tenure on the geriatric ward stretched over a decade, marked by a facade of friendliness and impeccable conduct. A compassionate figure, she would routinely take evening strolls around the ward, engaging in conversations that offered solace to both patients and staff alike. However, the benevolent aura surrounding her began to unravel after a fateful brain operation in 1976, setting in motion a series of unsettling whispers.

Rumors, like shadows, crept through the hallowed halls of the hospital. Whispers suggested that the nun, once regarded for her piety, had forged an unconventional connection, a clandestine, purportedly lesbian relationship with a fellow religious sister. Their shared dwelling outside the convent walls and frequent visits to upscale restaurants painted a stark contrast to the austere life they had vowed to lead. In an unexpected departure from her solemn vows, Sister Godfrieda acquired a motorcycle, an emblem of defiance, as she cruised through the town of Wetteren, forsaking the traditional nun's habit with each wave to curious onlookers.

Yet, the most damning accusation against the nun, who had pledged a life of poverty, was the inexplicable abundance of funds at her disposal. The whispers intensified when, in the solitary hours of the evening, she indulged in the delicate meat of boiled lobsters in the ward's kitchen, a decadent act that did not escape the watchful eyes of the staff.

Behind the closed curtains of the ward, the secrets grew darker. A bloodied urinary catheter and a pair of rubber gloves emerged as grim artifacts beside one patient. An elderly woman, grappling with illness, bore witness to mysterious bruising. The arrival of Sister Godfrieda in her distinctive sturdy shoes, cloaked in a long white habit, became an omen, and missing medications only deepened the sense of unease. Whispers transformed into gasps as peculiar sounds emanated from behind the bed curtains, preceding the inexplicable demise of those who found themselves in the shadows of the nun's presence.

The staff, burdened by the weight of their concerns, had long voiced their grievances to the hospital administration. Accusations of verbal abuse, with Sister Godfrieda hurling derogatory terms like 'whore' and 'nervous wreck' at patients, formed a litany of complaints. Tales of a laundry basket thrown and a shocking act of public urination painted a picture at odds with the serene nun they once knew.

Despite their desperate pleas, the hospital's management chose to turn a blind eye. The ward staff, undeterred, clandestinely documented the unsettling occurrences surrounding the deaths of their patients. The tipping point came when one nursing assistant, grappling with a moral dilemma, confided her suspicions to the ward doctor. To her surprise, he harbored similar doubts but remained inert, opting not to confront the haunting allegations.

With the toll of unexplained deaths reaching a disturbing crescendo, the nursing assistant gathered courage to elevate her concerns. Seeking refuge in the chairman of the Public Center for Social Welfare, the guardian overseeing the hospital, she anticipated validation. Instead, she faced a stern admonishment, warned to silence her suspicions in the absence of concrete evidence or face the unsettling prospect of departure.

Confrontation

In the hallowed halls of the hospital, Sister Godfrieda's serene presence masked a clandestine storm brewing beneath the surface. Whispers of conspiracy reaching her ears, and she, ever vigilant, believed a sinister plot was unfurling against her. As the evening cast shadows on the dimly lit corridors, she confronted the whistleblower, issuing veiled threats.

The nursing assistant, undeterred by the intimidation, found herself once again on the doorstep of the chairman of the Public Center for Social Welfare at dawn. His alarm resonated with the higher echelons, prompting an intervention. Sister Godfrieda was send to the family doctor, who forces her to report sick.

Beneath the surface of this seemingly devout nun lurked a darker truth. An addiction had ensnared Sister Godfrieda, a consequence of the morphine injections administered post-brain surgery. A swift transfer to a detoxification clinic followed, where the routine of her days was punctuated by visits from a loyal confidant, her lesbian housemate, a teacher.

Emerging from the shadows of addiction, the nun returned, surprising all, reintegrating into the geriatric ward. Where the death toll had mirrored the ebb and flow of ordinary life within the medical enclave. Unbeknownst to her peers, a daring few confronted Sister Godfrieda, armed with a damning list of patients who had met their demise under suspicious circumstances.

In a burst of anger and denial, the nun fled the ward, only to collide with the arms of the Royal Gendarmerie, a twist of fate that would unravel the layers of deception shrouding Sister Godfrieda's seemingly tranquil existence.

Cover Up

Cause in the intricate web of concealment, the whistleblower, aside from confiding in the chairman of the Public Center for Social Welfare, also sought out a physician within the same institution in February 1978, unraveling the enigma surrounding the peculiar deaths. Swiftly and resolutely, the doctor, recognizing the gravity of the situation, takes the courageous step of alerting the authorities. Behind closed doors, an intricate investigation begins as they meticulously amass evidence, discreetly passing it into the hands of the Royal Gendarmerie, laying the foundation for a thorough investigation.

As the investigative lens delves into the labyrinth of duty rosters and patient records, a shadow of suspicion envelops Sister Godfrieda. The nun, seemingly cloaked in piety, is apprehended, and with startling immediacy, she confesses to administering a fatal dose of insulin to three unsuspecting patients. At 44 she is, despite her rehabilitation, still addicted to morphine. The facade of the once exemplary nun unravels within the confines of pretrial detention, exposing a disquieting disturbance within. Her roommate, the teacher, secretly provided her with the narcotic during her stay in rehab, adding a layer of complexity to the unfolding narrative.

Simultaneously, the graves exhume secrets, revealing a macabre truth. The forensic pathologist's discerning eye can only pinpoint an excess of insulin in three unfortunate souls, while the rest, whether cremated or decomposed beyond recognition, making toxicological research impossible.

The verdict of Sister Godfrieda of the court in Dendermonde is that of complete mental incapacity, consigning her to an indefinite stay in a psychiatric institution. The brain surgery performed two years prior is seen as the reason for her aberrant conduct.

The exact tally of victims remains shrouded in speculation, and the timeline of the somber chapter when lives were extinguished remains elusive. The presumed count, veering closer to thirty than the proven three murders, paints a harrowing picture.

In the shadows of ecclesiastical influence, the representative of the hospital's Board of Directors and the steadfast ward staff disclose a disconcerting truth. The Catholic Church orchestrated a carefully crafted veil of silence, strategically concealing details such as the clandestine lesbian relationship, opulent lifestyle, and the nun's substantial financial holdings. A resounding silence echoed from the congregation of the Holy Apostolines of Saint Joseph, allegedly manipulating circumstances to declare Sister Godfrieda mentally unsound without the scrutiny of a trial.

Softly

Despite her disturbed mind, the nun is able to unveil a chilling revelation of why she poisoned her patients. Especially killing the sick who were a nuisance during her night shift and who kept her from her well-deserved rest. She feebly extends an apology, attempting to cloak her malevolence with the thin excuse that the lethal insulin was administered 'softly,' sparing her victims from agony. Skepticism looms large, for the cruel grasp of an overdose on insulin is known to unleash torment beyond imagination.

The Gendarmerie, in a stern declaration, castigates her actions. The nun's maleficence knows no bounds as she strips fragile, elderly souls of their meager fortunes and cherished trinkets, a financial plundering to satiate her insatiable appetite for opulence and succumb to the clutches of morphine. Amid vehement denials of murder for monetary gain, she confesses having read in the newspaper about the Dutch nurse Frans H, who also killed his patients with insulin.

Post sojourn within the confines of a psychiatric bastion, she retraces her steps to the convent. Where she silently succumbs to the passage of time suffering of dementia, finely laid to rest at the venerable age of eighty-six, after a discreet church service, in the sacred enclave of the nuns.

Sister Godfrieda's enigmatic tale has been etched into cinematic lore, brought to life in the celluloid realm as "Killer Nun" (1978), featuring the iconic Swedish film siren Anita Ekberg, a captivating symbol of allure from the tumultuous 1950s.

3.

Fear of failure and overconfidence: a fatal combination

Reinhard B., Germany, 1975

Initial Problems

In the chilling winds of mid-October 1975, Rheinfelden in the southwest of Germany saw the grand inauguration of the Kreis Hospital, a serene haven nestled in lush greenery. A line of flags danced on the lawn, caught in the sinister whispers of the October wind. The festive atmosphere, adorned with the melodies of a brass band and the graceful twirls of dancers in lederhosen and dresses with puffed sleeves, masked the brewing storm within.

Half a year prior, the hospital operated in a trial run, a facade of freshly painted walls and sparkling equipment. Patients trickled through its doors, and the first operations are carried out. There are numerous initial problems, especially in intensive care, amid the gleaming medical apparatus. A critical absence haunted the corridors, the lack of a departmental physician cast shadows on the seamless functioning of the hospital. But the true drama unfolded in the interpersonal dynamics, a dark dance between the authoritarian supervisor and the male nurse, Reinhard B.

Accusations of arrogance echoed through the sterile hallways as the supervisor clashed with Reinhard B. Her demands to temper his dominating presence during meetings fell on deaf ears. He, in turn, found her admonishments unforgivable, a sentiment that would shape the trajectory of events to come. To sidestep her influence, Reinhard plunged himself into the shadows of night shifts and prior to the official opening, the supervisor was transferred. The winds of change blew ominously through the white halls, carrying with them the untold secrets of Rheinfelden.

Panic

In the halls of healing, the purpose of a healthcare institution is as clear as day, a sanctuary where the ailing are meant to find solace and recovery. Yet, in the heart of the newly christened Kreis Hospital's intensive care unit, a chilling paradox unfolds. Instead of tales of triumph over illness, a silent specter of death begins to weave its shadowy narrative.

The ominous prologue commences within the initial 32 days since the hospital's grand opening, ten unsuspecting souls, seeking solace in recovery, died. A sense of foreboding settles over the medical staff as doctors and nurses hastily convene. Something is awry, a discordant note in the symphony of healing. The twilight state preceding these untimely deaths clashes with the medications administered, casting a haunting veil of uncertainty. An overdose suspicion flickers briefly, but the majority of the cases remain shrouded in enigma.

In the subsequent three days, the macabre dance of fate quickens its pace, reaching a crescendo on December 20. Three souls are silently escorted to the mortuary, one after another, leaving a disconcerting trail of unanswered questions. Doctors, armed with stethoscopes and files, plunge into the labyrinth of medical records, desperate for a flicker of enlightenment. Yet, the elusive clue remains elusive. A grim pattern emerges, a sinister triad of symptoms: vomiting, labored breaths, and hearts careening out of control while blood pressure plummets. Despite the valiant efforts of the resuscitation team, does not govern the patient's heart muscle by the appropriate means. Laboratory revelations unveil a toxic cocktail of heart medication.

As doubt looms heavy, the doctors reluctantly pen natural-death declarations. However, after the demise of three more souls, a chilling epiphany takes root, foul play taints the sterile corridors of the hospital. The alarm is sounded, and the management hastily summons the enforcers of justice. In a clandestine ballet, detectives, cloaked in the sterile white of medical practitioners, stealthily navigate the labyrinth of leads. The medicine cabinet, usually a bastion of healing, stands betrayed, revealing a conspicuous absence of a potent medication. Amidst the ongoing care for the remaining patients, the nurses find themselves on the precipice of anxiety. A vigilant sister unearths a clandestine graveyard of empty vials of heart medication in the dustbin. Sixty-three discarded vessels bear silent testimony to a sinister design.

Among the absent caretakers on this ominous day is Reinhard, a figure now immersed in the realm of Morpheus. Whether his rest is tranquil or haunted by the echoes of events is an open question. At the strike of 11:00 p.m. on December 21, as he endeavors to embrace the night shift, the long arm of justice seizes him. The investigators, shrouded in the guise of authority, assert that he alone was the nocturnal witness to the unfolding tragedy.

Accidentally?

Under supervision Reinhard exits the ward, slips into the elevator, and emerges in the lobby where the ominous presence of a police car awaits, stationed like a sentinel.

Within the confines of the police station, Reinhard is subjected to scrutiny. His bag, a repository of secrets, spills its contents onto the table, an assortment of medicine bottles and strips, predominantly tranquilizers and sleeping pills. The suspect, now an unwilling player in a high-stakes drama, engages in a torrent of words, extolling the virtues of the ward under the watchful eye of a new supervisor. In a confessional stream, he admits taking matters into his own hands, administering medications to patients, and, in a whisper, hints at the possibility of accidental overindulgence. His foot incessantly taps, and trembling hands betray an inner turmoil, leaving the detectives to ponder the mystery before them.

Born in 1948 as the sole son in a family of five sisters, Reinhard is raised as the Benjamin, a doted-upon and compliant boy, steeped in religious devotion. In moments of tension, particularly during headaches, he grapples with absences, brief epileptic seizures that usher him into a realm of fleeting unconsciousness. Early on, he seeks refuge in painkillers for his headaches, retreating to the sanctuary of his bed.

On brighter days, he revels in the childhood fantasy of playing doctor, adorned in a makeshift white coat, brandishing a faux stethoscope and a toy syringe, orchestrating imaginary healings for his entire family. Despite physical ailments, he perseveres through high school, nurturing dreams of evolving into a male nurse.

His journey begins with the commencement of his nursing training, where he resides on campus but clings to the familiarity of home during his rare days off. A likable enigma to his peers, Reinhard remains elusive, his inner world shielded from prying eyes.

At the age of twenty-one, he claims his diploma with pride, surrounded by the cheers of his father, mother, and five sisters. Post-ceremony, jubilation is accompanied by Schnaps and cheesecake.

Reinhard sets his sights on a dermatology clinic and from academia to the practicalities of the medical world heralds a newfound phase, one where he hopes to be taken seriously.

Yet, as the years unfold, no subtle transformation occurs expect that he retreats into increasing isolation, a solitary figure navigating the labyrinth of his existence. The absence of romantic entanglements is inconsequential; he finds solace in solitary walks and the rhythmic embrace of swimming, a ritual observed twice weekly without deviation.

Non-Committal

In Reinhard's twenty-fourth year, his world is shadowed by the death of his father, and a storm of health issues descends upon him. The specter of insomnia looms larger, and his appetite fades into obscurity. Sweating profusely, trembling, he becomes a frequent absentee, grappling with the encroaching malaise. Over a span of nine months, he visits his doctor forty times, getting cocktails of painkillers and tranquillizers prescribed. At the tender age of twenty-five, he undergoes scrutiny in a neurological department, yet no ailment is unearthed, and Reinhard resumes his place in the realm of daily toil.

Fast forward two years from the passing of his father, and a tempest brews within the walls of the dermatology clinic. Accusations surface, alleging unsanctioned pill administration to patients. The nursing staff, including Reinhard, staunchly defends their professionalism, refusing to be easily implicated. Despite the absence of a designated culprit, tension tightens its grip around Reinhard. Days unfold in a haze, and nights withhold the solace of sleep. The breaking point arrives as he collapses, ushering him into a five-week sojourn within the corridors of a psychiatric department. There, psychiatrists weave a diagnosis of a schizoid personality and obsessive-compulsive disorders, painting a portrait of a young man entwined in compulsions, shunning social connections, hypersensitive, yearning for a stable haven, and oscillating between realms of inferiority and overestimation.

Upon release from the psychiatric crucible, the psychiatrist's counsel prescribes a path of less demanding work and the embrace of psychotherapeutic intervention. A somewhat noncommittal recommendation, for there exists no oversight to ensure its adherence.

Reinhard, choosing the familiar confines of home, turns his back on the dermatology clinic. In time, he self-proclaims readiness for the job market, securing positions only to face dismissal on grounds of incompetence.

Then, the summer of 1975 unveils the stage for the impending Kreis Hospital in Rheinfelden. A clamor for staff obliterates the meticulous checking of references, paving Reinhard's swift entry. Despite an offer to lead the intensive care unit, he demurs, opting for the role of an executive nurse. On September 1, 1975, six weeks before the official inauguration.

Beyond the initial clash with his supervisor, Reinhard crafts an impressive facade. Colleagues warm up to him, swiftly entrusting him with the intricate responsibility of daily patient care. His commitment knows no bounds, as he graces the ward well before the clock ticks the start of his shift. Patients, if conscious, willingly seek solace in his assistance, and Reinhard consistently carves out time for a fleeting chat, portraying an unwavering willingness to go above and beyond.

Yet, when the pressure intensifies, a common spectacle in the high-stakes realm of intensive care, then, as predicted, he fails. Ventilators and medication calculations elude his grasp despite earnest endeavors. In the throes of critical moments, he appears frozen, a tableau of helplessness.

In a bid to conceal his inadequacies, Reinhard embellishes his medical prowess, donning an air of insolence. The damning phrase, "Lets give up on this patient," escapes his lips, marking just one of many missteps. Colleagues, in later revelations, suggest that Reinhard, from the onset of the sinister murders, withdraws into an increasing state of isolation. In brief, Reinhard finds himself ensnared in a familiar web of predicaments.

What only surfaces in the shadows of time is that the male nurse meticulously tends to death records before his victims embark on their eternal journey. Facing investigators, he tenders an apology, asserting that he pre-filled paperwork in a fog of absentmindedness. During the final, futilely attempt at resuscitation, an IV bottle slips from his grip as he exits the patient's room. Detectives unravel a significant medication order placed at the same juncture: one hundred ampoules on Monday, followed by another fifty of the same drug on Tuesday. Two days hence, as investigators scrutinize the case, the entire stock has vanished, leaving behind a chilling trail of whispers and deceit.

Motionless

In the eerie stillness surrounding Reinhard, the crescendo of evidence linking him to the deadly epidemic swells to an undeniable roar, leading to his official arrest. He pens a statement, only to retract it the following day, citing coercive pressure during his interrogation. As the shadow of serial murders by healthcare staff looms, an extensive prelude to the investigation unfolds.

Fast forward to 1977, two years after the chilling revelations first came to light, and Reinhard B. stands trial in the solemn halls of the Freiburg court. The prosecutor, swift and unyielding, orchestrates a courtroom spectacle. Alongside the customary testimonies, visual aids take center stage. A meticulous model of the intensive care unit rests on a vertical tabletop, becoming a visual compass for the unfolding narrative. As statements unfold, the court clerk gestures towards the victims' beds, unraveling the spatial dynamics, the distance between the medication cabinet and the ailing patient, the watchful gaze of Nurse A and Doctor B. observing his suspicious actions.

In the hallowed courtroom, Reinhard faces charges for seven murders, a sinister tally that likely conceals more hidden horrors. The inaugural victim, confined to the intensive care unit after a harrowing bowel surgery, struggled through a labyrinthine postoperative recovery. Witnesses among fellow patients recall the fateful moments, an ominous silhouette with a filled syringe, bed curtains drawn closed three-quarters of an hour before the inevitable departure of the patient from the realm of the living.

The second heart-wrenching episode unfolded in the recovery of a man who had undergone laparoscopic surgery and was improving. In a statement later retracted by Reinhard, he claimed to have administered a double dose of a heart stimulant. Undeterred in his choice of a lethal substance, the nurse consistently delivered the same medication.

When the wife of the subsequent victim visited her ailing husband, he drew his final breath just as Reinhard lingered by the bedside. In a confession, Reinhard B. acknowledged administering two ampoules to the man.

The fourth victim, a cancer patient, unexpectedly departed four days after a determination in the operating room that further surgery held no merit. Similar to the fifth and sixth victims, Reinhard B. took on the role of the sole caregiver for these patients. The last two, both women, died shortly after their arrival in the intensive care unit. In the case of the seventh victim, a colleague noticed the suspect lingering unusually long beside her bed. According to his later retracted statement, Reinhard administered three ampoules to this patient. Autopsies for all the accused murders revealed a toxic amount of heart medication.

In the defendant's seat, the male nurse, with his slender shoulders and large, dark-rimmed glasses, remains motionless, hands folded in his lap. Unwavering and devoid of emotion on his face, he responds to the questions.

The prosecutor's steadfast conviction of the defendant's guilt becomes apparent from the outset of the trial. Reinhard B. purposefully drew a lethal overdose of medication into the syringe in the medicine room, administering the toxic substance to his victims with the sole intention of causing their demise. Despite the seemingly absurd nature of the act, the prosecutor concedes that the motive remains speculative. It may sound implausible, but the only explanation at hand is that the defendant, driven by ambition, adamantly refused to acknowledge his inadequacies in performing his duties and, out of a sense of helplessness, administered the fatal overdoses.

Cerebral Abnormality

In the intricate labyrinth of legal proceedings, the revelations from psychological and psychiatric evaluations cast significant shadows. But before plunging into the depths of that matter, let's journey back to the year 1975, the onset of Reinhard B.'s macabre practices, when scrutinizing serious criminals for potential brain abnormalities was considered unequivocally 'wrong.' It was the era of the Dutch 'Buikhuisen affair' in 1979, a time when criminologist Wouter Buikhuisen faced vehement criticism from the left-wing for his attempt to explore the roots of criminal behavior. He believed in the potential predisposition of individuals to criminal behavior based on biological traits, such as diverse reactions to stress or the influence of testosterone, stood in stark contrast to conventional wisdom. The journey from that controversial period to the present day has witnessed significant strides in brain research, providing unmistakable evidence supporting Buikhuisen's theories. The illuminating work of authors A. Moir and D. Jessel in *Born Criminals: A Fascinating Quest for the Biological Origin of Violence and Crime* (1995) firmly establishes the nexus between brain abnormalities and criminal behavior, echoing the profound implications revealed in Chapter 2, where the Belgian nun Godfrieda turned to murder following the removal of a brain tumor.

Now, returning to the outcome of Reinhard's psychological and psychiatric examination. According to the comprehensive report, his actions find a potential explanation in his schizoid personality. The tumultuous inception on the ward stripped away essential external stability, thrusting him into tasks that surpassed his mental capacity, teetering on the edge of debility. This left the suspect, whose self-worth was intricately tied to his role, grappling with an insurmountable predicament. To navigate this, he resorted to constructing an unrealistic self-image, blurring the boundary between reality and delusion, and succumbing solely to inner impulses steering him towards malevolent actions.

The conundrum of how an individual with intellectual disabilities managed to uphold the role of a nurse for an extended period captivates Reinhard's legal counsel, adding another layer of intrigue to this complex tale.

Procedural Flaws

In the unfolding legal drama, the defense takes center stage, unraveling the tapestry of evidence for a myriad of reasons. Their narrative unveils conspicuous flaws in the intricate workings of the dedicated intensive care unit. Casting blame upon the supervisor, they argue she allowed the nurse to tread beyond his capacities, overlooking the inflated self-confidence that veiled his subpar performance. The stage for an unsettling number of unexplained deaths was set in a recently inaugurated department struggling to meet standard benchmarks. Communication among physicians and other disciplines stumbled in inadequacies, and the staff found themselves navigating a landscape of insufficient training. A troubling lack of control loomed over medication orders; any nurse could wield the pharmacy without the ink of a doctor's signature, leaving a cloud of ambiguity over the delivered substances.

Further intensifying their defense, the legal team questions the evidentiary foundation for manslaughter. They postulate that the extraordinary cluster of deaths might be no more than a sinister coincidence, arguing the absence of clear intent on the part of their client. The determination of a toxic dose during autopsy, crucial to their case, was restricted to the narrow window within a few days after death. However, for eleven patients who succumbed shortly before the spike in deaths under analogous conditions, this window had already elapsed. Even within the permissible timeframe of six autopsies, the presence of the substance fails to furnish irrefutable proof. The defense articulates three key points: a lack of a direct link between the substance and the cause of death, an absence of evidence proving intentional administration of an overdose by their client, and an inability of expert witnesses to precisely quantify the fatal medication dosage.

The specialist from the Freiburg Institute of Forensic Medicine adds an unsettling layer of uncertainty, asserting that it cannot be definitively ruled out that the 66-year-old victim succumbed to an advanced gastric carcinoma after the laparoscopic surgery. In a perplexing twist, the prosecutor, in his indictment, hesitates on the brink of labeling the incident involving the 63-year-old patient as attempted murder. The fatal heart attack apparently defies confirmation through the lens of the presumed overdose. The cause of death for the final victim, aged 67, is ambiguously attributed to a massive toxic concentration, leaving an air of mystery hanging over the courtroom.

In addition, the defense asserts the imperative consideration of their client's mental state by the court. Should it be proven that he is accountable for the epidemic of deaths, they argue that his actions were rooted in a state of rational and emotional decompensation, consistent with a schizoid personality, characterized by a distinct decline in comprehension regarding measure and number.

In their final plea, the defense contends that the suspect should be acquitted, attributing this proposition to grievous errors committed during the initial police interrogation. The relentless questioning persisted for seven consecutive hours under the harsh glare of intense lights. Law enforcement officers concede to attempting to extract a confession from the suspect, dangling the prospect of mitigating circumstances and psychiatric treatment. Faced with resistance, the suspect was incessantly branded a murderer, accompanied by threats to involve 'older, less understanding officers' willing to employ harsher interrogation methods. Subsequently, under duress, the client confessed, only to retract it the following day.

Grounded in the use of unauthorized and coercive interrogation methods, the judge issues a verdict of acquittal. However, two years later, in 1980, Reinhard B. is ultimately convicted on appeal. The presiding judge, relying on the same psychological and psychiatric examination, deems him fully accountable. The judge finds the manifestations of fleeting psychoses, where the line between reality and delusion blurs, to be unconvincing. The nurse intentionally administered a lethal dose, fully cognizant of its fatal consequences. Despite not being the brightest, his theoretical knowledge extended sufficiently to anticipate the outcomes of his actions. Consequently, he is sentenced to seven years of imprisonment: one year for each murder, and a lifelong professional ban.

Turning the pages to the next chapter, we linger in Germany, leaping forward. In 2006, a 54-year-old nurse is arrested in Berlin. During her pretrial detention, sharing a televised interview, reminiscing about her childhood experiences wandering through her parents' home with a Red Cross kit at the tender age of five. Similar to Reinhard, she harbored a desire to assist people from an early age. Yet, the perplexing question persists: Why do serial killers in healthcare opt to do precisely the opposite?

4.

The outcasted woman

Irene Becker, Germany, 2006

The Interview

In the shadow of her conviction, Irene Becker's tale unfolds like a chilling narrative, a twisted saga that sends shivers down the spine. The camera sweeps across a seemingly innocuous setting, a room adorned with the relics of a life led astray. Neatly made bed and a modest desk, posters of Che Guevara and Martin Luther King, icons that stand as silent witnesses to a woman's descent into infamy. On a bookshelf the famous German author Hermann Hesse and the equally famous French philosopher Simone de Beauvoir, with some snapshots of a private secretary-type woman leaning against a tree trunk. Wearing a light-colored jacket, fashionable sunglasses on top of her hair. In another a tanned backpacker, with a handkerchief tied sportily around her head, jeans and sneakers.

Norbert Sigmund, the tenacious journalist, steps into the fray in the spring of 2007, armed with questions and an unyielding determination to unravel the mystery shrouding Irene's malevolent actions. Accused and having confessed to the unforgivable crime of administering fatal doses of medication to unsuspecting patients. By the time the exposé hits the airwaves that fateful summer, Irene is already consigned to the annals of criminal history.

As the program unfolds, a defiant 54-year-old Irene emerges, head held high, her countenance a blend of defiance and bitterness. The camera captures her piercing gaze as she confesses to a dearth of visitors, family long gone, her only solace found in the company of a friend who visits twice a week. A casual mention of the hospital director's visit raises eyebrows, as Irene nonchalantly apologizes for the pandemonium she has wrought.

When pressed to explain her macabre decision kill to patients, Irene, a woman of paradoxes, pauses before delivering an unsettling rationale: 'Everyone should be able to exhale their last breath on their own, without the help of a ventilator', again looking straight into the lens.

The interviewer, unrelenting in his pursuit of truth, probes her views on the fifth commandment 'Thou shalt not kill.' Irene, unmoved by the weight of her deeds, dissects the concept of 'death' with an unsettling detachment. She broadens the interpretation of the Ten Commandments, arguing that she didn't extinguish lives but merely curtailed their suffering. To her, it was a duty, administering fatal doses of medication, a twisted act of mercy, and a responsibility she bears willingly.

As Irene grapples with the consequences of her actions, a silver thread of faith weaves through her narrative. In her moments of despair, she finds solace in the embrace of God, seeking refuge in the pews of the church she frequents. A portrait emerges of a woman, both condemned and redeemed by her beliefs, a paradoxical figure in the annals of crime and punishment.

In the unsettling chronicles of those dubbed 'angels of death,' the initial foray into the abyss began with the publication of a chilling tome in 1998. The maestro behind this exploration is none other than the German psychiatrist and psychotherapist, Professor Karl Heinz Beine, hailing from the enigmatic University of Witten-Herdecke. His treatise, *Sehen, Hören und Schweigen* (See, Hear, and Be Silent), delves into the morbid labyrinth of 28 serial murders within the confines of care institutions.

As the echoes of his groundbreaking work reverberated, a subsequent chapter emerged in the form of another book *Krankentötungen in Kliniken und Heimen: Aufdecken und Verhindern* (Hospital Killings in Clinics and Homes: Uncover and Prevent). Professor Beine, now a key player, was summoned as an expert witness in the judicial drama surrounding nurse Irene Becker. His reflections on the televised encounter unravel a disturbing psychology.

In the shadows of these narratives, a common thread weaves through the profiles of these malevolent figures. Many of them harbor altruistic dreams from their youth, aspiring to assist the vulnerable, yet the recognition usually fails to materialize.

The convicted, in a perverse self-assurance, believes she fulfills the wishes of her patients. Yet, the truth lies in the darker recesses, it's an intricate dance around her own anguish. Her empathy with the victim's agony becomes a mirror reflecting her own unbearable suffering. The act of killing, a twisted catharsis, a 'self-discharge,' akin to the release observed in 'ordinary' serial killers after each murderous episode.

Professor Beine's analysis unravels the immense pressure cocooning these perpetrators in their earthly hell. A pressure manageable only as long as the semblance of control is maintained. But, like a tautly stretched wire, it's a matter of time before the strain becomes unbearable, and the need to strike again becomes an inevitable crescendo.

The interviewer, seeking the elusive truth, poses the question about Irene's relief post-administering the fatal doses. Craftily, she deflects, asserting her patients suffered no pain. A chilling revelation follows, a tacit admission that echoes through the corridors of malevolence. 'But don't think I'm the only one who thinks this way.' When confronted about others silencing their patients permanently, her nonchalant reply encapsulates the chilling banality of her actions, 'Well, I'm not that special, you know.'

The Psychiatrist

In the hushed corridors of justice, where the echoes of a woman's life reverberate through the annals of a court case, the haunting narrative of Irene Becker unfurls like the delicate pages of a psychological thriller. As the players step into the spotlight, the forensic psychiatrist emerges as the first storyteller, peeling back layers of Irene's existence, revealing a tapestry woven with darkness and redemption.

It all begins during Irene's pretrial detention, a period punctuated by five confidential conversations with the psychiatrist. Within those guarded confessions lies the haunting tale of Mrs. Becker's genesis, a journey marked by the cold embrace of an unloving family, childhood health issues, and the lonely shadows of a timid, quiet childhood. Seeking refuge, she flees into the sanctum of nursing with the Catholic order sisters, a cocoon of protection that sets the stage for her transformation into a stern, devout woman.

The narrative unfurls further, revealing Irene's odyssey through the Jewish Hospital in Berlin. A marriage devoid of offspring accompanies her ascent in the medical hierarchy, as she navigates a labyrinth of professional success tinged with interpersonal discord. Nineteen years of service culminate in a devastating crescendo as the management, weary of her tirades and defiance, demands her resignation. The taste of humiliation is bitter, a wound that drives her to the precipice of her own unraveling, seeking refuge in the hands of professional healers.

But every descent holds the promise of a rise, and Irene's redemption finds its stage at the Charité Hospital, the grandeur of the cardiac intensive care unit becomes the backdrop of her resurgence. Within those sterile walls, she rebuilds, finding solace in her work and the appreciation of her peers. A seasoned healer, Mrs. Becker does not flinch from the abyss of caring for the dying. On the contrary, she seeks out the most severe cases, oblivious to the chilling fact that death becomes an uninvited companion to those under her watch.

In her eight-year tenure at Charité Hospital, Mrs. Becker's life takes a harrowing turn when her husband becomes enamored with a much younger woman. The blow strikes her as a profound humiliation, setting the stage for a painful divorce process that unravels the threads of a thirty-year marriage deemed irreparable by 2005. The wounds suffered by this narcissistic woman, wounded in self-esteem, plunge her into the abyss of depression. The loss of her husband, a fundamental pillar of her existence, triggers a transformation where weakness and helplessness are masked by an artificially inflated self-esteem, a precarious facade to buoy herself up.

After a period of rebuilding, Mrs. Becker manages to regain some semblance of normalcy. She revamps her home and embarks on distant travels. The psychiatrist speculates that her heightened self-esteem may breed resentment toward the suffering she witnesses on the ward. Perhaps she believes that if doctors won't end the patients' torment, she should take matters into her own hands, not out of hatred for the patients, but a decision to no longer passively witness their agony.

When questioned about her feelings during the murders, Irene expresses only emptiness. In her eyes, it wasn't about murder; the lives of artificially sustained, terminally ill individuals held no value. She struggles to articulate why she intervened in their impending demise.

The psychiatrist delves into the nexus between her actions and her faith. Mrs. Becker proposes altering 'Thou shalt not kill' to 'Thou shalt not harm', arguing against needlessly prolonging the lives of terminal patients.

Did she act on God's orders? Mrs. Becker vehemently denies it, asserting she was merely a servant called to 'help' patients. The psychiatrist refrains from labeling her a monster, attributing her actions to a blend of personality traits and the turmoil of divorce. Her imbalance, he concludes, led to grave consequences as she projected her incapacity and anger onto those whose fates she determined.

Karl Heinz Beine introduces a grim coincidence, four days before intentionally eliminating a patient at Charité Hospital, Mrs. Becker dresses as an angel at a summer festival. He also notes her disconcerting behavior during the trial. Commendations from superiors evoke tears of joy, however, when listening to the suffering of the bereaved, showing no emotion.

The courtroom becomes a stage where tragedy, psychology, and a chilling narrative converge.

The Staff

In the hushed corridors of the hospital, where whispers of end-of-life discussions linger, the staff grapples with a daunting reluctance. Only under the persistent prodding of detectives during interrogations do they unveil the unsettling narrative that unfolds in the wake of nurse Irene's enigmatic presence. Like a silent storm gathering strength, their accounts reveal a shift in the seasoned nurse's demeanor, leaving an indelible mark on the ward.

End-of-life talks were commonplace among the staff, yet they recall no extremist views from Nurse Irene. She, like her peers, stood firm against the senseless prolongation of lives, earning a reputation as an experienced, competent, and dedicated professional willing to go the extra mile. However, a recent transformation in her conduct had cast a shadow over the once-respected figure. A cacophony of loud singing and shrill whistling echoed through the corridors, an incessant presence that grated on the nerves of all who encountered it. The staff hesitated to voice their discontent, well aware of nurse Irene's penchant for fierce reactions to criticism. The exact moment of this behavioral shift eludes consensus, perhaps drowned in the tumult of her divorce-induced stress.

Yet, as the curtain of time unfurled, Irene's actions turned from peculiar to outright unacceptable. Rough and abrasive, she snapped at patients as if the weight of the world rested squarely on her shoulders. In the chilling aftermath of death, laughter replaced empathy. A confession surfaced during a conversation with the supervisor, admitting having behaved aggressively. Even when presented with an offer to ease her workload temporarily, she vehemently declined.

The descent into darkness reached a critical juncture seven months before the arrest, it all escalated. Nurse Irene slapped a confused woman who had smeared herself with feces, and two months later, a similar incident occurred.

Colleagues reported these distressing incidents to the supervisor, who assured them of intervention. However, when the wheels of justice finally turned, no action had been taken against the errant nurse. The climax came in late November 2005 when nurse Irene, in the presence of a colleague, attempted to extinguish a life with a nonchalant injection of a potent painkiller, without order nor justification. The patient ceased to breathe, and only swift action from another nurse, urgently summoning a doctor, saved a life hanging by a thread. Shockingly, the doctor, when confronted with the report of this life-threatening incident, chose to turn a deaf ear.

The aftermath of these events casts a lingering shadow over the staff. They grapple with a profound sense of responsibility, haunted by the question of whether their silence allowed the nightmare to escalate unchecked. In the silence of the hospital corridors, where duty and dread intertwine, the untold tale of nurse Irene's transformation unfolds, leaving the staff haunted by echoes, partly feeling responsible for not raising the alarm earlier.

In the shadowed corridors of guilt, one male nurse bears the weight of an unsettling truth. Seven weeks before the inevitable shackles of justice ensnared nurse Irene, she wielded authority over the care of a 77-year-old soul tethered to terminal illness, a man whose ceaseless moans echoed through the sterile walls. Overheard in a chilling decree, Irene demanded an end to the tormented groans. Against the sanctioned accord with the doctor, the male nurse bore witness as Irene, with a calculated audacity, plunged a full syringe into the suffering patient, ushering him abruptly into the realm of the departed. Unsettled, he retrieved the discarded ampoules from the refuse, only to be met with a profound shock. The gravity of such a damning secret proved too immense for solitary confinement, and under the cloak of confidentiality, he unraveled the tale to two trusted confidants. When he went on holiday, he brooded groggily there on Spain's Costa del Sol, the weight of knowledge sinking into the sand beneath him. Later, he discovered that one colleague had breached the sacred pact upon hearing a doctor jest about another soul slipping away during nurse Irene's watch. Even the physician displayed an eerie lack of alarm. Since that moment, the colleague assumed the vigilant role, scrutinizing nurse Irene's every move. Despite returning from vacation, the nurse hesitated to broadcast his suspicions. A decade of shared life-saving endeavors with Irene stood as an insurmountable barrier against betrayal. In hindsight, regret clings to him like a remorseful shadow, for in the wake of the moaning man's demise, three more lives succumbed to the sinister machinations.

Others among the ranks step forward, bearing witness to a symphony of disturbing testimonies. A mere week before nurse Irene's descent into infamy, a peculiar episode unfolded. In the company of the patient's husband, Irene administered a fatal injection to a relatively young woman, her heart already tethered to the precipice of demise. Despite the woman's fervent desire for a homebound departure, an ambulance awaited her summons. The sudden demise cloaked itself in an enigma, leaving the onlookers to murmur amongst themselves.

A departmental doctor steps into the morose spotlight, unveiling his unsettling encounter with nurse Irene. Amidst a prolonged resuscitation effort, discord erupted between the two. Irene dismissed the doctor's endeavors as futile, advocating for the cessation of the ventilator's rhythmic hum. Post-resuscitation, she turned to a young doctor, questioning the sanctity of life, challenging the divine order itself. To her, the act of resuscitation was an affront to the Almighty's will.

The Prosecutor

In the theater of justice, the prosecutor unfurls a narrative woven with the sinister threads of Mrs. Becker's alleged deeds. A macabre tale unfolds, spanning the dark corridors of a hospital where life should be preserved, not extinguished. Between June 2005 and October 2006, eight lives stood at the precipice of Mrs. Becker's intervention, souls ensnared in the fragile realm between existence and the inevitable embrace of natural death. To her, the ebb and flow of life were forces that demanded her interference, wielding an authority akin to an omnipotent force. Without a physician's mandate, she would administer a potent elixir of lethal medication, ushering unsuspecting patients into the abyss.

The overture commences with a 66-year-old man, a frail figure lying on the precipice of mortality. As doctors feverishly attempt to breathe life into him, Mrs. Becker, a spectral figure in the medical drama, introduces a perilous dosage of a blood pressure-lowering agent. The physicians, unbeknownst to the lethal intervention, persist in their futile efforts. In a mere seven minutes, the patient succumbs, a mere pawn in Mrs. Becker's sinister chess game. The symphony of death continues with a 71-year-old man, subjected to an abnormal dose of a painkiller. The man's pulse, though feeble, clings to existence. The suspect hastily leaving the scene. Mrs. Becker becomes the architect of his untimely end.

The third movement unfolds with a 79-year-old man, a survivor of numerous surgical battles. In the twilight hours before his demise, coherence lingers, only to be abruptly extinguished without warning. Amidst the futile efforts of resuscitation, Mrs. Becker, like a puppeteer pulling strings, administers a lethal cocktail of injection fluid. In whispered confessions to a colleague, she explicitly declares she has injected 'everything.' A 66-year-old man becomes the fourth victim, succumbing swiftly to an excessive dose of anesthesia.

Approximately seven weeks before the final curtain of justice falls, Mrs. Becker defies the doctor's mandate, administering two fatal injections to a 77-year-old patient already resigned to the twilight of treatment. The sixth victim emerges, the only woman in the malevolent gallery of Mrs. Becker's crimes. A 48-year-old patient, supposed to return home to embrace the final chapter, falls victim to an overdose of a blood pressure-lowering agent. The husband, left to cradle the lifeless form of his wife, becomes an unwitting witness to the horrors orchestrated by Mrs. Becker. In the aftermath of this cruel spectacle, two more men are sacrificed at the altar of her sinister machinations.

The prosecutor, amidst the tapestry of horrors, refrains from connecting Irene's divorce to the transformation of her behavior. Yet, in the shadowed corners of speculation, one cannot help but wonder, does Irene's choice of victims, predominantly men, bear the scars of the humiliations suffered when her husband callously traded her for a younger counterpart? And does the lone woman in this ghastly narrative meet her demise as an unwitting witness to the intimate connection she once cherished, a cruel reminder of Irene's own lost love since her divorce? The courtroom, now a stage for justice, awaits the unfolding of this grim drama, where the lines between motive and madness blur into a chilling crescendo.

The Judge

Irene Becker's defense attorney struggles to move beyond portraying his client as a warm-blooded, highly intelligent, and clever woman who simply sought to shorten the suffering of patients. He emphasizes that if those in charge on the ward had responded more effectively, the number of victims would have remained limited.

The judge however, delves into the intricacies of the case with a meticulous and expansive perspective. He grapples with the complexity of a legal narrative woven from the fabric of 130 scrutinized deaths. Compounded by the peculiar setting where demise is an inherent facet, the presence of medications that could yield dire consequences in the wrong hands adds layers of complication. Rarely has he borne witness to crimes so insidiously committed. In his discerning gaze, that is why he believes that Mrs. Becker is particularly guilty, for he believes that every life, regardless of its brevity, holds inherent worth and merits protection.

The judge unmasks Mrs. Becker's transgressions, asserting that she, with a brazen defiance of the sanctity of life, established her own laws. These laws, far from compassionate, dictated the cold-blooded murder of terminally ill souls. He dismisses any notion of euthanasia, pointing out the absence of evidence indicating her actions were prompted by the plea of the patient or their family. The proof of overdoses found in the bodies of some victims solidifies, in his discerning view, the heinous nature of these murders.

In the solemn chambers of justice, the gavel falls with a resolute decree. Mrs. Becker is condemned to a life behind bars for five counts of murder and one count of attempted murder, coupled with the charge of assault. Yet, amidst the echoes of justice, there is a nuanced refrain. The third charge concerning the 79-year-old man and the fifth charge concerning the 77-year-old man remain unproven, leading to Mrs. Becker's acquittal due to a glaring lack of evidence. The courtroom, once a stage for the grim theater of Irene Becker's deeds, now bears the solemnity of a judgment rendered, a chapter closed, but the shadows of her actions linger in the corridors of legal history.

The Hospital

In the turbulent aftermath of Irene B.'s arrest on October 4, 2006, the corridors of the cardiac intensive care unit and the executive suites of Charité Hospital resonate with lingering echoes of culpability. As their former employee faces stern judgment, the judge extends the long arm of the law to those leaders who turned a blind eye to the mistreatment and, shockingly, the outright murder of patients under their charge. Interrogations of colleagues resurface, each inquiry probing the unsettling question: Why did they remain silent? The resounding truth emerges, no one, absolutely no one, entertained the possibility that a trusted fellow nurse could harbor the sinister intent to deliberately extinguish the lives of vulnerable patients.

Soon after, the hospital finds itself entangled in the web of accountability spun by one bereaved family member seeking justice for his father. A son's grief becomes a potent force as it unravels a tale where a colleague of the convicted nurse, aware that something nefarious was afoot, withholds crucial evidence before nonchalantly embarking on a vacation.

A week preceding nurse Irene's arrest, a clandestine meeting unfolds among the departmental doctor, the ward doctor, and the supervisor. Suspicion simmers, prompting them to share their concerns with the elusive head of the clinic. Despite the intensive care unit basking in the glory of being recently recognized as the best department, boasting the lowest cost per patient, and with an implicit expectation of unwavering commitment from its staff, the head of the clinic remains shrouded in unreachability for an entire week. Later, in the courtroom's hallowed confines, he attempts to contest his conspicuous absence.

The judge, wielding the power of righteous judgment, metes out a directive as a punitive measure against the hospital. The duty entrusted to medical and nursing staff, he asserts, is to safeguard the well-being of patients. Consequently, a commission must be established to dissect the labyrinth of missed opportunities, culminating in a comprehensive report that outlines policies designed to forestall any recurrence of such horrific events. As a symbolic act of accountability, the head of the intensive care unit is summarily dismissed, echoing the solemn gravity of the judgment resonating through the halls of Charité Hospital.

5.

Passion with fatal consequences

Kristen Gilbert, United States, 1989

In Love

In the military hospital in Northampton, protocol dictates the presence of a security guard during every crisis situation, including those on Ward C, the intensive care unit. A measure intended to keep onlookers, such as visiting patients, at bay. The guard in question doesn't mind this at all; in fact, he relishes it. As the medical and nursing staff work tirelessly to save lives, he stands by, reminiscent of a character from a Hollywood film, *Nurse Falls for Security Guard,* with his thumbs hooked behind his belt. Cause what does that one nurse want?

For six years now, Kristen has been a stalwart member of the evening shift, known as a respected nurse, though one doctor would later scoffingly refer to her as a walking medical manual. Yet, even he couldn't deny her prowess during resuscitations. With fervor, she clambers onto the hospital bed, barking commands as she pumps the patient's chest. And could it, could it be, in the process of the act, being unaware her skirt riding up so high that her underwear is visible? Strangely she seems to attracts trouble, as almost all crises occur during her shifts. Afterwards, graciously accepting compliments from the security guard. And as the number of crises increases, seeking his company more and more. For by August 1995, the butterflies in her stomach have transformed into a tempest, she can't resist brushing against him, feigning accidental closeness. Whether the patient was saved is not her concern, but she remembers vividly if he was smiling back.

By chance, they cross paths in the parking lot, leading one thing to another. But there's a problem: the attractive ICU nurse is married.

Spiraling Downwards

In the eerie calm of the Strickland household, Kristen Heather emerged as the beacon of hope, the eldest daughter destined for greatness. But behind the façade of impeccable curtains and meticulously manicured lawns lay a darker truth, concealed from prying eyes. Seven years later, a younger sister would join the family, but the tranquil exterior still belied the tumult roiling within.

Kristen possessed the allure of youth, with her slender frame and cascading locks, capturing the attention of her peers effortlessly. Yet, beneath her charming facade lurked also a shadowy undercurrent, a propensity for deceit and manipulation that would unravel the fragile fabric of her existence.

It began innocently enough, a petty theft here, a lie there, weaving a web of deception that ensnared all who dared to trust her. As she embarked on a career in caregiving, her actions bordered on the macabre, a chilling disregard for the lives entrusted to her care.

But Kristen craved attention and sympathy, inventing stories making people feel sorry for her. She was good at manipulating others' emotions to get what she wanted.

And then there was Glenn, the unsuspecting suitor drawn into her web of deceit. Their courtship was a whirlwind of movie dates and shared meals, masking the darkness lurking beneath the surface. Yet, as their union solidified, so too did Kristen's grip on reality loosen, her demands escalating to terrifying extremes.

For eight years, Kristen remained Mrs. Gilbert. Three years after the birth of their first son, announcements once again graced the mail. The family now boasted two boys. Kristen, by then, was already working at the military hospital, seemingly embodying both the model housewife and the caring nurse simultaneously.

Throughout the eight years of her marriage, all the family's cats, dogs, and guinea pigs met their demise under suspicious circumstances. The marriage bore the heavy burden of her lies and deceit. For Glenn, the final straw came when her affair with the security guard came to light. Kristen attempted to poison Glenn, left the children with him, and closed the door behind her for good.

She rented her own place and constantly spoke ill of her ex-husband. And although the security guard would admit to having had thrilling encounters with her, he soon saw the dark side of his plaything. Provocatively, she demanded he choose between her and his cat, and as a joke, he chose the poor creature. She then fed the cat a poisonous morsel, refused to take the dying animal to the vet, and falsely claimed to the neighbor that she had performed mouth-to-mouth resuscitation, on the cat that was.

When she claimed to be pregnant, the man was shocked. She became distressed, curling up in the fetal position, murmuring: 'I haven't done anything. You have to believe me.'

What on earth was she talking about? Kristen began banging her head against the wall so violently that he dialed the emergency number and had her admitted to a psychiatric hospital, where she was diagnosed as 'manic-depressive'. When he collected her toiletries from home, he found an empty ampoule in her bathroom cabinet. Meanwhile, Glenn had filed for divorce.

Minor Flaw

Let's journey back into the chilling motives of serial predators lurking within the confines of healthcare facilities. Research delves into the heart of darkness, revealing that among the myriad tragedies unfolding within these sterile walls, it is those tethered to the most critical units, like the harrowing confines of an intensive care ward, who bear the brunt of malevolence. Here, patients lie ensnared in their beds, their very existence dependent on the life-giving drips that weave through their veins, oblivious to the surreptitious injections that may seal their fate. In this realm where death lurks as an ever-present specter, a rise in mortality rates passes by unnoticed, camouflaged amidst the cacophony of medical urgency.

It may sound callous, but participating in a resuscitation effort evokes heroic feelings, especially among healthcare providers with low self-esteem. Consequently, some serial killers actively seek out the 'rush of saving lives', even if it means putting the patient in a life-threatening condition, such as administering harmful medications. To the murderer, the patient not surviving the resuscitation is merely a minor flaw.

From the moment Kristen stepped foot into her role, an unsettling pattern began to emerge. Just a year into her employment, one of the ward physicians abruptly barred her from tending to his patients, citing a suspiciously high mortality rate under her care. Even the observant receptionist couldn't help but notice Kristen's frequent presence during resuscitations and patient passings. Concerned, she dared to raise the alarm with management, only to find herself accused of malicious gossip.

Yet, as the legal saga unfolded, the same management vehemently denied any such conversation with the receptionist, casting a chilling shadow over the institution's integrity. More troubling still was the revelation that these heightened incidents of resuscitation had slipped through the cracks of those entrusted with oversight, despite their prominent roles on the Medical Emergency Committee.

Initially shrouded in silence, Kristen's colleagues eventually found their voices, peeling back the layers of secrecy to expose the unsettling reality lurking within the hospital's walls.

Shoulder Trouble

It was February 1996 when Kristen's life took yet another unexpected turn. Six months into her clandestine affair, she finds herself sidelined at home with a shoulder injury, Curiously, as Kristen nursed her physical ailment, the frequency of resuscitations on the ward returned to a semblance of normalcy, a fact not lost on her vigilant colleagues. Sensing a troubling correlation, they raised the alarm once more, their voices finally reaching the ears of hospital authorities, who swiftly involved the police.

As suspicion cast its shadow upon Kristen, her colleagues recalled a disturbing series of events from the preceding year. In the throes of her blossoming infatuation, vials of crucial medication mysteriously disappeared from the ward, coinciding with an unsettling rise in resuscitation cases. Kristen's demeanor, once compassionate, had transformed into something altogether callous. Her laughter echoed through the halls in the presence of grieving families, a chilling testament to her newfound indifference to human suffering.

With the investigation looming, the security guard ensnared in Kristen's web of affection grew increasingly uneasy. Sensing impending trouble, he hastily severed ties with her, hoping to distance himself from the looming storm. Meanwhile, Kristen, now stripped of her job and desperate to evade interrogation, resorted to drastic measures. Blocking her former lover's driveway with her car, she embarked on a desperate bid for attention, culminating in a harrowing series of suicide attempts.

Her actions, as puzzling as they were chilling, led to her repeated admissions to psychiatric care. Psychiatrists, grappling with the enigma of Kristen's psyche, diagnosed her with an insatiable craving for attention, fueled by a dangerous penchant for risk-taking. Yet, amidst the darkness of her deeds, one thing remained abundantly clear, her story was far from over.

In the meticulous search of Kristen's apartment, investigators stumbled upon a chilling revelation, a table meticulously listing potential witnesses to her sinister deeds. Their scrutiny extended to the homes of her ex-husband, Glenn, and her children, yielding a stolen handbook on poisons, its pages dog-eared to the sections outlining the substances she had allegedly administered.

Come October 1996, when the suspect nurse was taken into custody, she vehemently refuted any wrongdoing. However, her behavior during interrogation painted a different picture. Rocking back and forth in her chair, a telltale sign of profound psychological distress or profound cognitive impairment, she deliberately misled investigators with false information. The toll of her confinement manifested physically, her once svelte frame now swollen from over a year in pretrial detention.

Yet, amidst her gluttony, Kristen found time for more sinister pursuits. Sending an anonymous bomb threat to the military hospital, where suspicion immediately fell upon her, seemed to evoke a perverse delight. Confiding in a friend, she admitted relishing the attention it garnered. Adding to the intrigue, she authored a manuscript detailing a murder mystery set within a state institution, featuring a protagonist eerily reminiscent of her own circumstances. When authorities confiscated the manuscript, Kristen brushed it off as mere fiction, but she wasn't the only healthcare serial killer to commit her crimes to paper.

In 1998, the story of French nurse Christine Malèvre sent chills down the spine of readers worldwide. Convicted of six heinous murders and suspected in a staggering 24 more, she delved into the depths of darkness with her memoir: *Mes aveaux* (1999). In its haunting pages, she unflinchingly recounted how her own pain seemed to evaporate as she extinguished the suffering of others. A bone-chilling parallel emerged with Genene Jones, the enigmatic figure at the heart of Chapter 12, who embarked on her own literary journey, though her narrative remained tragically incomplete.

This unsettling phenomenon of chronicling one's own crimes stretches beyond the extraordinary to touch the lives of even the most 'ordinary' of serial killers. Psychologically dissected, it's theorized that through the act of writing, perpetrators traverse back through the corridors of their dark deeds, finding a perverse pleasure in revisiting their atrocities, albeit in the safety of the written word.

Meanwhile, the saga of Kristen Gilbert unfolded in January 1998 when she faced formal charges of four premeditated murders, three attempted murders, and forgery. Despite the gravity of the accusations, she was granted bail, trading the confines of a jail cell for the watchful eyes of electronic surveillance at her parents' home. However, her relentless pursuit of various individuals, including her former lover, drew the ire of law enforcement. In a bid to quell her reign of terror, the police took the drastic step of temporarily severing her lifeline to the outside world, her phone, leaving her isolated and awaiting her fate in a chilling limbo.

Numbers

Getting a suspected serial killer in healthcare behind bars is a devilish task. Each piece of evidence, each witness testimony, is a thread to be followed, leading deeper into the murky depths of deception and despair. And when the final tally is made, when the truth is laid bare in stark numerical form, the chilling reality emerges.

To start with, in Kristen Gilbert's case, there are 18 months of pre-trial investigation, during which 70 witnesses are heard. During her seven-year tenure at the military hospital, there are a total of 350 deaths on Ward C. Just under half of these are pre-resuscitated, with Kristen 'discovering' the cardiac arrests in a quarter of cases, where patients were improving and whose hearts were functioning properly beforehand. The rest of the staff 'discover' the cardiac arrests in the other quarter of cases, where their life-threatening condition was preceded by a deterioration in their overall health. In the 4 months before Kristen's sick leave, there are 30 resuscitations during her late shift; 23 patients die. In the 4 months thereafter, while Kristen is sitting at home on the couch, there are only four deaths and two resuscitations during the day, evening, and night shifts combined.

Gaps in medication delivery are discovered on Ward C. It is subsequently determined that the pharmacy delivered 115 vials of cardiac stimulants in

1995 and 1996, which, apart from Kristen, no one ever used. The trial itself will last 5 months. After presenting 200 pieces of evidence, hundreds of hours of witness testimony, and more than 250 motions, the jury can begin its deliberation. The jury then takes another 12 days to reach a decision. And all of this results in 10,000 pages of court records, including medical files and police reports.

Death Penalty?

As Kristen glides into the courtroom six years post-arrest, flanked by vigilant guards, her presence is a stark contrast to the woman once known for her caring demeanor. She's visibly slimmer, adorned in a tailored suit, her lips painted with meticulous precision.

The expert witness, a statistician, takes the stand, his analysis painting a chilling picture. The odds of Kristen coincidentally stumbling upon so many patients teetering on the brink of death, considering her part-time schedule, are deemed one in a million. This renders the possibility of her having no involvement in the resuscitations and high mortality rate astronomically small. A forensic pathologist, after extensive study, concludes that all victims died from acute medication poisoning with a cardiac stimulant. According to the cardiologist, there's a distinction between a natural death and sudden cardiac death. In a natural death, the patient succumbs to their illness before the heart stops. In sudden cardiac death, the heart ceases without warning.

Then, the ex-husband and relatives of the defendant take the stand. Glenn testifies against his wife. She had confessed to him that she administered overdoses of medication to patients, necessitating resuscitation. She sarcastically remarked that those who died simply received a bit too much. Later, she attempted to retract her words, claiming it was just a joke.

Glenn appeals to the court, considering their two children, to refrain from imposing the death penalty. Kristen, who has had little or no personal contact with her sons since leaving home, has written the boys at least 300 letters during her pretrial detention.

The father of the defendant and both grandmothers plead with the court for understanding. The execution of Kristen would also devastate their lives.

The death penalty, a relic of some American states, hangs precariously over Kristen's fate like the mythical sword of Damocles. Though the state of Massachusetts itself abstains from such punishment, her transgressions within the confines of a military hospital, under federal jurisdiction, thrust her into the perilous realm of capital punishment.

But even in this case, the evidence dangles by a thread. Errors in the calculation of the medication overdose in the exhumed bodies leave only circumstantial evidence.

As the gavel falls, the verdict darkens the air with finality. Kristen, once a healer entrusted with lives, is now branded with the weight of three counts of premeditated murder, one count of manslaughter, and two counts of attempted murder. The sentence: four life terms without the possibility of parole, coupled with two twenty-year sentences for the attempted murders. A fate both harsh and merciful, as her family members, though relieved, cannot escape the somber realization of what might have been. According to the judge, she truly deserves the death penalty for the calculated manner in which she murdered her victims.

Upon hearing the verdict, Kristen bows her head, her shoulders shaking. Her lawyer initially files an appeal but withdraws it because Kristen doesn't want to risk ending up on death row.

Why?

What compels Kristen, in her relentless pursuit of attention, to seek a spotlight where she can perform? The psychological intricacies explored by Vaknin and Rangelovska in their book *Malignant Self-love, Narcissism Revisited* (2005) shed light on this perplexing phenomenon. They posit that a narcissist's insatiable craving for validation drives them to extreme lengths, even if it means embracing negative attention over insignificance. Thus, the media circus surrounding her conviction for atrocious crimes might serve as a twisted form of affirmation for Kristen. Engineering medical emergencies to play the role of savior, she delves into a world of heroic fantasies where she reigns supreme. Researchers have coined various terms to capture this behavior: *Super Nurse, Code Blue Junkie, Professional Heroism, Hero Complex*, and *Power Seekers*.

Kristen's attorney vehemently denies that his client is a murderer. He contends that the crimes occurred under immense mental and emotional strain. With no evidence of intent and lacking direct proof, he argues for her acquittal.

However, the fires that blazed through Ward C. between 1990 and 1993 add another layer of darkness to Kristen's narrative. Among the flames, Kristen was often the first responder, hailed as a hero for her efforts in extinguishing the infernos. Yet, beneath the accolades lies a chilling truth, a pattern of arson intertwined with her other deadly deeds.

In the annals of crime, Kristen is not alone in her deadly fascination with fire. Alongside her, other Health Care Serial Killers have been drawn to its destructive allure, their actions leaving scars on both flesh and psyche. Charles Cullen from Chapter 21 tries to set fire in the bathroom and kill himself; the Belgian nurse Kurt Dobbelaere from chapter 20, just like nurse Michaela Giersberg from the next chapter, sets his house on fire.

6.

The girl who was supposed to be a boy

Michaela Giersberg, Duitsland, 2003

Inferno

In the tranquil countryside near the quaint West German town of Wachtberg, a serene farmhouse stood as a beacon of rustic charm. However, on that fateful day in May 2005, the tranquility shattered, engulfed in flames that would leave scars both physical and emotional.

Amidst the idyllic scenery, a woman sat alone in her car, her thoughts consumed by a turmoil of despair. With a flick of her hand, she cast a smoldering cigarette out the window. Creating a spark who found its mark in a heap of loose straw, setting ablaze the very foundation of the farmhouse.

As the inferno raged, consuming everything in its path, a family's history crumbled along with the burning timbers. Frantic shouts pierced the air as the elderly parents narrowly escaped the engulfing flames, their ancestral home reduced to a smoldering ruin.

About a kilometer away, as the crow flies, in May 2005, the supervisor of the woman behind the wheel sat waiting in her office, unaware of the impending storm brewing in her employee's life. A year prior, one of her caregivers had casually mentioned the looming shadow of chemotherapy, a necessary evil to combat a brain tumor. But there was more beneath the surface, a hidden turmoil stemming from familial scars, dragging her into the depths of therapy.

Nestled in the quaint town of Wachtberg, just south of Bonn, lies the Altenstift-Limbach nursing home, promising solace to its 130 residents, some grappling with the relentless grip of dementia. The idyllic complex, with its quaint red-roofed cottages encircling the main building atop the hill, held the promise of a peaceful twilight for the elderly. However, what followed next would shatter this illusion.

While anxiously awaiting updates on her caregiver's chemotherapy schedule, the supervisor received an unexpected missive from the psychotherapist, imploring her employee to provide extra support. Weeks later, a note of gratitude followed, attributing the caregiver's resilience to the supervisor's care. But it was the cryptic mention of postponing chemotherapy that raised suspicion.

Intrigued, the supervisor delved deeper, only to discover a shocking revelation: the psychotherapist claimed ignorance of the correspondence. Was it possible that the caregiver herself had penned the letter, weaving a web of deception amidst her own struggles? The truth, as always, lay buried beneath layers of deceit, waiting to be unearthed.

With a keen eye for detail, the supervisor pieced together a puzzle fraught with sinister implications. Whispers of concern from a vigilant colleague hinted at a pattern too unsettling to ignore. Each time during the shift of the nursing aide in question, a remarkable number of residents breathed their last, as if orchestrated by an unseen hand.

The supervisor's heart raced as she laid the files of the deceased beside the duty roster, tracing the chilling synchronicity of their departures. It was a revelation that left her breathless, a realization that something far more sinister lurked beneath the surface.

Summoning her courage, the supervisor confronted her employee, seeking answers amidst the unsettling silence that followed. But as the hours passed and the truth remained elusive, a startling headline in the morning paper shook her to the core.

From the quiet corridors of a nursing home to the charred remains of a farmhouse, the threads of mystery intertwine in a narrative that grips the reader from start to finish. As the pieces fall into place.

Correspondence

In the span of a mere week, the unassuming walls of the police station witnessed a scene straight out of a psychological thriller. The interrogation room, a stage for the unraveling of a chilling confession, held the 27-year-old nursing aide, her figure betraying a mix of defiance and vulnerability.

At first, she clung to denial like a lifeline, vehemently refuting any involvement in the deaths of four residents. But as the pressure mounted, her facade crumbled. With tear-filled eyes and a trembling voice, she began to unravel a tale of horror.

Amidst prayers and hymns, she admitted to smothering three helpless souls with a pillow, a macabre ritual that left no room for mercy. Her confession, delivered with a mix of remorse and detachment, chilled the room to its core.

But the horror didn't end there. In a revelation that sent shockwaves through the room, she confessed to six more murders, each one a testament to the darkness that lurked within her soul.

As the investigators probed deeper, she clung to her confession.

In a courtroom drama that rivaled the most gripping of true crime tales, Michaela stood before the judge, her fate hanging in the balance. Despite her attempts to recant her confession, the judge saw through her facade, recognizing the depths of her guilt.

Declared fully accountable by the court-appointed psychiatrist, Michaela's attempt to escape the consequences of her actions fell on deaf ears. In the end, her story served as a haunting reminder of the darkness that can lurk within the most unexpected of places.

Michaela Giersberg found herself in the grip of the law, her once unassuming life now a focal point of legal scrutiny. After an exhaustive examination of all 261 deaths during her six-year tenure, she faced charges of deliberate acts resulting in the demise of nine elderly women afflicted with dementia, aged between 79 and 93.

During her preliminary incarceration, a troubling disarray permeated the demeanor of the once-esteemed caregiver. In a poignant letter addressed to her parents, she bared her soul: 'Please, don't forsake me. Throughout my existence, I've strived relentlessly to embody your cherished vision of "Michel," the son capable of shouldering the farm's burdens. At nine, a stark realization dawned, I was no daughter, but a son. With mother pregnant with her next child, her pleas echoed for the much-longed-for son. Instead, I gained a sister. With the onset of my menses, disarray engulfed me. My physique assumed the guise of femininity, yet my heart yearned for masculinity. Early in the morning, my grandfather abused me sexually in the meadow behind the shed. Asking me: "Why do they call you Michel, anyway? I'll show you what a girl you are!" Which let me questioning for years, was I Michel, or was I Michaela? But to everyone, I was just a stubborn child, and no one bothered to listen.'

Angel of Death

A haunting moniker emerges in the media of The Angel of Death of Wachtberg. Behind this chilling alias lurks an accused nursing aide, her story unfolding in the hallowed halls of the Bonn court. It's a swift procession, beginning its macabre dance in January 2006, a date etched in the annals of swift justice. Thirty-seven witnesses take the stand, their testimonies like threads in a tapestry, weaving truth from deception.

Enter the stage, Michaela's former comrades and supervisor. They paint a portrait of a dedicated soul, revered by residents and their kin. Michaela's devotion knew no bounds, extending beyond duty into the realms of compassion. Even in her leisure, she walked among the elderly, a beacon of solace guiding them to church.

But behind this facade lies a darker narrative, reminiscent of my earlier explorations into what I've termed the 'Mother Teresa Syndrome.' Frans H. and Godfrieda, both beckoned by a divine call to the convent, yet this inclination towards self-sacrifice isn't exclusive to those who take vows. It's a trait shared by those who walk the line between caregiver and malefactor, their dedication cloaking their sinister designs within the sanctity of healthcare.

Michaela's peers held her in high esteem, marveling at her unwavering cheerfulness despite personal strife. She was more than a mere caregiver; she was a pillar of her community, donning multiple hats, city council member, carnival reveler, and horn player in the local brass band.

And yet, amidst the accolades, whispers of suspicion lingered. The supervisor, at first blinded by Michaela's seemingly impeccable care, now grapples with doubts. Were the deaths mere coincidences, or were they orchestrated by the very hands entrusted with healing? The defense seeks answers, and the supervisor, her voice trembling, reluctantly confirms Michaela's mastery in her craft, a proficiency that earned her a place of honor in the labyrinthine corridors of the psychogeriatric ward.

In the realm where light meets darkness, where caregivers morph into perpetrators, Michaela's tale stands as a cautionary testament to the enigmatic allure of the Serial Killer in Healthcare.

Oath of Secrecy

Before the courtroom drama unfolded, Michaela absolved her two psychotherapists and her trusted physician from the bonds of confidentiality.

Since December 2001, Michaela had been ensnared in the tangled web of psychotherapy. Her initial therapist lamented the scant progress made during their sessions. Delving into the murky waters of incest only dredged up agonizing memories. By early 2005, when the therapist insisted on confronting her father, Michaela abruptly halted the sessions. Now, the therapist hears whispers from the prosecutor's corner suggesting that the alleged abuses by either her grandfather or father were but phantoms.

Michaela's GP had been a stalwart presence since April 2002. No matter what ailment was discussed, the specter of abuse always loomed large. Even she now grapples with the realization that the tales of her father or grandfather's malfeasance were nothing but figments of imagination. Yes, she had encouraged her patient to confront her father about the alleged incest, yet Michaela remained obstinate, even when reminded of the peril faced by her younger sister. The patient's refusal stemmed from her father's chilling threat of releasing damning video footage of the atrocities. In a moment of courtroom drama, the judge's incredulity pierced the air: 'How could a father wield such a video, portraying himself as the villain, to coerce his own daughter?' The doctor could only falter in response.

Until just before she was taken into custody, Michaela had attended 35 sessions with a second psychotherapist. Despite persistent encouragement, she adamantly refused to confront her father or to live independently. Here, as in other aspects of her life, the haunting memories of past abuse consumed her, particularly her reluctance to take over the family farm. Following her pregnancy, it is alleged that her father accompanied her to an abortion clinic. Michaela had revealed to this therapist a letter from her mother that hinted at her awareness of the incest. The therapist, with caution, affirmed that there was no basis to question the validity of these events.

Emotionless

In the courtroom, the defendant is painted as a habitual liar, a label vehemently contested by Michaela. She argues fiercely, claiming the prosecutor spins natural deaths into tales of murder. A forensic psychiatrist enters the fray, portraying the woman as a dynamic, goal-oriented personality. Yet amidst her apparent vigor, Michaela harbors traits wholly incongruent with her profession. 'Mrs. Giersberg lacks emotion to such an extent that she cannot forge any meaningful emotional bonds. She embodies traits of egocentricity, recklessness, and stubbornness. But above all, she harbors a deep-seated rejection of her own gender, feeling unattractive and shunned.'

The defense seizes upon this psychological profile, advocating vehemently for an acquittal on grounds of mental incapacity. They argue that their client harbored dreams of inheriting her father's farm, dreams tragically unrealized. The relentless abuse inflicted by her grandfather left her scarred, cultivating an insidious sense of inferiority. In her quest for safeguard, Michaela weaved a web of lies, exchanging untruths for attention and consolation. The lawyer underscores the addictive nature of her craving for attention. With her fabricated brain tumor, Michaela's sole desire was to occupy the spotlight.

Self-Pity

After a series of futile attempts by the prosecution to present concrete evidence, the Bonn court reaches its decisive verdict. Admitting to the absence of direct proof, the court acknowledges the challenges in the case. Despite signs of violence found in the autopsies of two female victims, all deaths were attributed to natural causes. Complicating matters further, the majority of victims had been cremated, potentially erasing crucial evidence. The defendant initially confessed to the murders only to later retract her statements, but her detailed accounts of suffocation, containing intimate details only known to the perpetrator, leave no doubt in the judge's mind regarding the veracity of her admissions.

Delving into the psyche of Michaela, her motivations become clearer. In her sole confession, she painted a portrait of herself as a compassionate soul, acting out of pity. She claimed to have ended the suffering of severely ill residents upon the urging of an inner voice. One victim, she recounted, had pleaded with her through their eyes, a plea she interpreted as a direct wish for death. Yet, in another chilling twist, she recounted how she callously allowed another victim to suffocate, incapable of expelling her own phlegm.

The scant presence of compassion becomes glaringly apparent from her comment about the troublesome, uncooperative women getting on her nerves. In fact, compassion isn't the apt descriptor here; as scientist Karl Heinz Beine suggests in Chapter 4, it's more about self-pity. He posits that these cases typically involve deeply insecure individuals grappling with long-standing, unresolved issues.

As per the court's ruling, the defendant meticulously and cruelly ended the lives of vulnerable elderly individuals between November 29, 2004, and April 24, 2005. Consequently, she's found guilty of four counts of murder, four of manslaughter, and death on demand. The potential number of victims may even surpass these figures, as suggested by the court physician at Uni-Klinik in Münster, who hints at the possibility of 'undiscovered' victims for every 'discovered' one. The charge of arson, however, is dismissed. When the judge delivers the verdict of a life sentence and a lifelong professional ban, Michaela breaks down in tears, burying her face in her hands.

In the realm of healthcare serial killers, administering a lethal injection is the modus operandi for most. Strangulation or suffocation, as seen in Michaela's case, is far less common. However, if we rewind the clock about twenty years, we uncover a chilling case where two American healthcare workers engaged in a bizarre game, resulting in the suffocation of six patients.

7.

Lethal liaison

Gwendolyn Gail Graham and Catherine May Wood, United States, 1986

Crossword Puzzle

In the quaint town of Grand Rapids, Michigan, a sinister tale of forbidden love and murderous desire unfolded in the halls of Alpine Manor nursing home. The year was 1986, and the protagonists were none other than Gwendolyn Gail Graham and Catherine May Wood, two seemingly ordinary nursing aides whose dark appetite led them down a path of depravity.

From the moment Gwen, a young and alluring 23-year-old, set foot in Alpine Manor, she captivated the attention of Cath, a formidable figure with a haunting allure. Their connection was instantaneous, a dangerous spark that ignited a whirlwind romance laced with deception and treachery.

As the nights grew longer, so did their sinister bond. Gwen and Cath, driven by their insatiable desires, orchestrated their shifts to coincide, ensuring they were always together during the twilight hours. Their nocturnal escapades were a dance of death and seduction, a twisted game played against the backdrop of the nursing home's dimly lit corridors.

But behind their facade of romance lay a chilling truth - Gwen's lust for power and control knew no bounds. In the cold grip of January 1987, she committed her first act of murder, targeting an unsuspecting Alzheimer's patient. With calculated precision, she silenced her victim, leaving behind no trace of her heinous crime.

As the body count rose, so did the stakes of their deadly game. Gwen and Cath reveled in their newfound freedom, their passion fueling a dangerous dance on the edge of sanity. But their reign of terror was short-lived, as whispers of suspicion began to circulate among the staff of Alpine Manor.

Lethal liaisons: the alpine manor tragedy unravels the harrowing tale of two lovers consumed by their darkest desires. Set against the backdrop of a serene nursing home, this chilling account exposes the depths of human depravity, where love becomes a lethal weapon and passion turns deadly.

In the chilling saga of their twisted partnership, their first sinister act solidifies a bond that transcends morality. With a vow as dark as the deeds they commit, they pledge their undying allegiance to each other through a macabre ritual - alternating murders to bind their fates together. Each victim becomes a macabre testament to their deadly union, whispered promises of 'Forever and one day' haunting the aftermath of their crimes.

As their tally of atrocities grows, so does their grotesque tally, marking their grim journey with a morbid scorecard reaching towards 'Forever and six days.' But even in their twisted games, there are lines they dare not cross. Cath's crossword-inspired scheme, attempting to rationalize their brutality, crumbles under the weight of their escalating violence. The notion of selective slaughter based on the letters of 'MURDER' proves futile, a fleeting whim abandoned after the second kill.

Their victims, mere pawns in their sordid game, suffer the cruel fate of their whims. Left to suffocate in the silence of their crimes, their screams silenced by the cold hand of death.

For Cath, the horror of their deeds lingers, a chilling reminder of the darkness lurking within. She recoils from the scene of their atrocities, her screams of terror echoing through the corridors of their twisted reality. Yet, in the safety of their home, Gwen and Cath revel in their depravity. Intoxicated by the scent of whiskey and the haze of hashish, they indulge in a dance of pain and pleasure, their bodies intertwined in a macabre celebration of their deadly desires.

Thank-You Note

In the shadows of the Alpine Manor nursing home, a sinister aura begins to permeate the air long before the truth is unveiled. Patients voice concerns more frequently, with one woman even screaming of attempted rape. Strange deaths cast a pall over the facility, like the unsettling demise of a resident found dead after a heated exchange with a nurse's aide, dismissed as a mere heart attack by the attending physician.

The day preceding the passing of a demented woman, her son notices telltale bruises adorning her frail frame. Staff explanations of accidental bumps clash with his mother's usual stillness in bed, raising unsettling questions.

Cath, a figure shrouded in mystery, whispers ominous threats to a wheelchair-bound patient, warning of dire consequences should he speak out again. The night supervisor grapples with the enigmatic duo, sensing an unsettling dynamic between them. Colleagues, only daring to voice their concerns in retrospect, paint a troubling portrait of Cath, a manipulative figure adept at weaving lies, with a penchant for control.

Cath's domestic life is far from idyllic, a stark contrast to societal norms. She shuns traditional roles, opting instead for the escapism of daytime dramas and the comfort of potato chips. Motherhood proves an ill fit, evidenced by her neglect of her daughter upon moving in with Gwen. The child's father, incensed by Cath's negligence, confronts her in a scene of drunken chaos, only to be met with violence from Gwen's hands while declarations of love for Cath hang heavy in the air. Yet, Gwen's affections are fleeting, quickly shifting to another. Cath, consumed by jealousy, retaliates with a brutal assault on her perceived rival, leaving a mark that goes beyond the physical.

In the wake of this chilling incident, four of the six murders unfold in a harrowing succession spanning just sixteen days. Each nefarious act is strategically executed on the eve of their scheduled days off, meticulously shrouded in deceit as the patient's condition is intentionally misrepresented to mask the true cause of death. The initial victim of this spree is discovered lying supine, a telltale rolled-up washcloth left conspicuously on her blanket. Oblivious to the sinister reality, the family, upon cremation, extends their gratitude to the staff for their purported care with a thank you note.

Barely a week later, the second patient succumbs under mysterious circumstances. A haunting scene unfolds as the victim's mouth hangs agape, the lower jaw unnaturally skewed to one side. Despite the alarming signs, the attending physician hastily attributes the demise to a heart attack. However, the deceased's shaken roommate, now haunted by fear, refuses to sleep in the dark.

The subsequent deaths, occurring within a single shift ten days later, paint a portrait of unrelenting horror. One victim is discovered lifeless in bed, devoid of any prior signs of deterioration, while the other is found with their right arm eerily wedged beneath their lifeless form.

Amidst this torrent of tragedy, two notable incidents cast an ominous shadow. A mysterious call from an unidentified staff member a week prior alarms the son of the fifth victim, urging him to rush to the hospital if he wishes to see his mother alive. Yet, upon arrival, he finds her alive and well, raising suspicions of foul play. The day preceding her murder, he observes ominous red marks adorning her nose and jawline, a chilling harbinger of the impending doom.

Gay

The atmosphere at Alpine Manor had taken a dark turn, with Gwen and Cath careening down a path of reckless behavior, punctuated by their twisted sense of humor. Their antics, once harmless pranks, now veered into disturbing territory as they hid under beds, startling unsuspecting colleagues, or played callous jokes on vulnerable patients.

As tensions simmered between the two, Gwen's refusal to sever ties with her new paramour only fueled Cath's growing aggression, leading to a volatile dynamic between the pair. When later faced with interrogation, Cath brazenly flipped the script, deflecting blame onto Gwen in a desperate bid to evade justice.

In a crescendo of depravity, their final crime unfolded nearly six weeks later, leaving a resident lifeless and her dentures discarded in the trash, a chilling testament to the depths of their depravity.

But behind the facade of Alpine Manor's cheerful exterior, chaos reigned within its walls. A revolving door of staff members, plagued by chronic understaffing, created an environment ripe for disorder. The discord spilled over into their personal lives, with the predominantly homosexual evening and night shift staff engaging in tumultuous relationships, earning the facility the moniker 'Gay Manor.'

As the turmoil escalated, residents bore witness to a breakdown in professionalism, with staff abandoning their duties to indulge in personal pursuits, while insults hurled at vulnerable residents further tarnished the institution's reputation. Amidst the chaos, a sense of foreboding loomed, signaling the unraveling of order within the once-harmonious walls of Alpine Manor.

Blind

Cath's relentless threats to expose their crimes echo in Gwen's ears until she's left with no choice but to show Cath the door. As Cath begrudgingly watches Gwen's new lover's belongings being carted out, a sense of bitter resignation settles over her.

In a curious twist, Cath's evaluation report at the nursing home paints a rosy picture following the demise of their relationship. Despite objections from the night supervisor, Cath earns a promotion to a coordinating nursing assistant. However, this promotion doesn't sit well with her colleagues, who soon become disgruntled by Cath's frequent absences due to alleged illness, resulting in a stern warning just a month after her elevation.

Meanwhile, Gwen and her roommate embark on a fresh start, severing ties and relocating. Despite the distance, Cath's torment continues unabated, her threats falling on deaf ears. Desperate for vindication, Cath resorts to betrayal, confiding in a colleague about Gwen's alleged acts of patient strangulation.

Amidst the turmoil, Cath finds solace in the familiar arms of her ex-husband, but a drunken confession unveils a startling revelation when Cath confesses the murders to him, plunging him into a state of bewildered shock. Months pass, and the weight of Cath's revelation gnaws at him until he finally seeks solace in therapy, where the therapist urges him to confront the truth and report the crimes.

In this harrowing account, reminiscent of the chilling narratives of serial murders in healthcare previously detailed, we're confronted with a disturbing reality: valuable time slips away before the heinous crimes come to light. Whistleblowers, motivated by a sense of duty, find themselves met with a deafening silence as their concerns are brushed aside and their complaints fall on deaf ears. A fellow caregiver, driven by suspicion and concern, dares to commit his thoughts to paper, only to have his written fears torn to shreds by the very hands of the head nurse.

Amidst the turmoil, the steadfast night supervisor emerges as a beacon of integrity, undeterred by the dismissive attitudes that surround her. Despite her earnest plea to stagger Cath and Gwen's shifts being summarily disregarded, she refuses to surrender to complacency. When she dares to speak out after a suspicious death, her expectation that Gwen would face consequences is met with bitter disappointment. Undeterred, she takes her concerns directly to the head of nursing, also to be met with a callous shrug and a dismissive wave of indifference.

Even the brazen boasts and unsettling behavior of the perpetrators fail to raise alarm bells. Despite their macabre confessions and the chilling displays of their 'trophies' including a sock from one of their victims, their audacious proclamations are met with disbelief and incredulity. It's a sobering reminder that even the most egregious warning signs can be overlooked in the face of institutional indifference and bureaucratic apathy.

Lassie

Gwen entered this world as her mother's third child, amidst a backdrop of transient homes and her father's sporadic employments on various farms. It wasn't until she was nine that their family finally found a semblance of stability.

Despite her affectionate nature, Gwen harbored an inexplicable aversion to sitting on anyone's lap. Her childhood memories were stained with the sight of her father pushing her mother's head in the flushing lavatory. An image that instilled in Gwen a lifelong fear of being drawn into rushing waters as punishment for any perceived misbehavior.

Gwen was thrust into farm life at an early age, even learning the gruesome task of pig castration from her father. But it was one particular event that scarred her psyche forever. After a session of unspeakable cruelty, her father coerced Gwen into shooting their beloved dog, Lassie, by the lake. This traumatic incident birthed within Gwen a deep-seated fear of vast bodies of water. She meticulously extracted Lassie's teeth from the lifeless body, preserving them in a macabre keepsake box and eventually displaying the skeletal remains in her room. Even upon her relocation to Grand Rapids, Gwen couldn't part with Lassie's bones, a haunting reminder of her past. Much like Michaela Giersberg from preceding accounts, Gwen hints at unspeakable harm inflicted upon being raped by her father, though the truth remains shrouded in ambiguity.

By the time she turned seventeen, her parents' union had crumbled, and Gwen's aspiration of becoming a veterinarian faded into obscurity. Instead, she found solace in the adrenaline rush of racing through city streets clad in leather motorcycle gear. However, her pursuits often led to perilous spills and grievous injuries. During a violent altercation, Gwen was rendered unconscious for two days by an adversary. Moreover, she terrorized her neighborhood with armed robberies and forged checks. It was around this tumultuous period, at the tender age of twenty, that she embarked on her first lesbian relationship.

After years of wandering, Gwen eventually found herself seeking employment in the very nursing home where a series of chilling murders would later unfold. Upon her departure a year later, the head of nursing extended a favorable recommendation to Gwen at a temp agency. Settling in a new town with her partner, she swiftly secured a position at a children's hospital. It was there, amidst the innocence of infancy, that Gwen casually mused to a colleague about the absurdity of a mother witnessing throwing her baby against the window. Cath, however, steadfastly maintains that her confession to the murders stemmed from a deep-seated fear that Gwen would perpetrate harm upon a child.

Connecting the Dots

Cath's upbringing was also far from ordinary. Raised in the very town where the unsettling events at the nursing home would later unfold, she endured a tumultuous childhood as the eldest among her siblings. She harbored resentment towards her mother, feeling overshadowed by her mother's affection for their dogs over her own children. Meanwhile, her father, marked by his experiences as a Vietnam veteran, enforced discipline with a heavy hand whenever he wasn't found at the local pub.

Assuming caretaker responsibilities for her younger siblings at a tender age, Cath struggled with the demands of nurturing, often resorting to physical and verbal aggression towards her siblings. Their home mirrored Gwen's, with constant turmoil leading to her parents' eventual separation. Despite Cath's academic prowess and remarkable memory, she found herself alienated by her peers due to her unpredictable demeanor.

It was during her high school years that Cath crossed paths with her future husband, culminating in a swift marriage following an unexpected pregnancy. By then, Cath battled with a profound sense of inferiority, exacerbated by her considerable weight of 150 kilograms. Plagued by occasional auditory hallucinations and fleeting thoughts of violence, she grappled with obsessive-compulsive tendencies, compulsively showering up to four times a day. Amidst these struggles, it was Gwen who offered Cath a glimmer of acceptance and affirmation, providing her with a newfound sense of allure and belonging that she had long yearned for.

In a scenario that seemed straight out of a twisted thriller, Glenn, Cath's ex-husband, arrives at the police station to divulge Cath's chilling confession. The officers are initially taken aback, suspecting a vendetta-driven accusation, but in early October 1988, they decide to extend an invitation to Cath for clarification. Without hesitation, Cath corroborates Glenn's account, painting a disturbing picture of Gwen as the mastermind behind the murders. Cath's explanation of her own involvement adds another layer of complexity; what began as a seemingly innocuous suggestion from Gwen soon spiraled into a nightmarish reality. Cath confesses to being Gwen's lookout during the heinous acts, admitting to finding a twisted thrill in the events unfolding before her.

There's an eerie detachment in Cath's demeanor, as if she's oblivious to the gravity of her actions. Even during the polygraph test, she remains oddly composed, offering compliments to the technician's friendly demeanor. Meanwhile, the investigative team, armed with mounting evidence, begins to connect the dots, suspecting foul play in six suspicious deaths.

As the tension escalates, Gwen, forewarned by Cath's threats, braces herself for the impending visit from detectives. Despite facing a barrage of questions, Gwen maintains her innocence, staunchly denying any involvement in the crimes. Nevertheless, she finds herself slapped with a work ban as law enforcement closes in, eventually leading to Cath's arrest followed by Gwen's.

Boredom

Despite Cath's admission, the investigation into the crimes proved to be lengthy and thorough. Additional autopsies were conducted on some of the bodies, but yielded little substantial evidence. The trial commenced in September 1989, as is customary in the American legal system, with a jury present.

During the trial proceedings, Cath confessed to her involvement in the murders. She revealed that the plan to suffocate patients was born out of sheer boredom. The first discussions of murder arose approximately four months after Gwen's employment began at Alpine Manor. Cath claimed that it was Gwen who proposed the idea of taking turns killing patients based on the letters MURDER. Their targets were chosen carefully, focusing on patients who were unable to communicate verbally, in case the murder attempts were unsuccessful. Cath accused her former partner of five attempted murders.

Throughout the trial, Cath displayed various emotions, occasionally covering her mouth in apparent shame while discussing the details of the murders. When a psychologist diagnosed her with a pronounced narcissistic personality, Cath broke down in tears. Testifying against Gwen ultimately resulted in Cath receiving a reduced sentence. Instead of facing life imprisonment, she was sentenced to twenty to forty years for manslaughter and conspiracy to commit murder, with the possibility of parole.

A mere week after Cath's conviction, Gwen found herself seated in the defendant's chair, facing the grim reality of six premeditated murder charges. With an air of defiance, she denied each accusation vehemently. Unlike Cath, who attempted to appease the interrogators with cooperation, Gwen's responses were curt, her demeanor aloof, as if the gravity of the questions failed to rouse any emotion in her. It seemed she was eager to retreat to the confines of her cell, unbothered by the weight of her impending judgment.

According to reports, Gwen was diagnosed with borderline personality disorder, navigating the world with a superficial and childlike understanding. Like Cath, she appeared devoid of self-worth, still yearning for the love she had never known. The only semblance of sensation she experienced was the searing pain of pressing cigarette butts against her skin. Evaluations painted a picture of a classic psychopath, one who sought increasingly risky behavior in search of release, devoid of any remorse or empathy. However, the intricacies of the original plan, devised during a casual crossword puzzle session to align with the six letters of MURDER, seemed incongruous with Gwen's limited imagination and emotional depth.

Relying solely on witness testimonies, Gwen was ultimately convicted of five counts of premeditated murder and conspiracy to commit murder. Stoically, she absorbed the verdict: five consecutive life sentences, devoid of any possibility for parole.

Partners in Crime

Even following Cath and Gwen's conviction, lingering questions persisted about their roles and influences in the gruesome crimes. Was Cath the callous mastermind, reveling in the infliction of pain, while Gwen was merely a manipulated accomplice coerced into carrying out Cath's sinister plans? Or did Gwen undergo a transformation under Cath's sway, becoming an unwitting instrument in a series of meticulously executed murders? The post-conviction behavior of both women only served to deepen the mystery surrounding Cath's true nature.

Despite her earlier claims of a troubled childhood, Cath emerged as a cunning manipulator within the prison walls, adept at pitting others against each other to serve her own ends. She cunningly shifted blame onto Gwen for crimes she purportedly committed, possibly out of vindictiveness or a desire to evade full accountability.

In stark contrast, Gwen maintained a stoic silence, steadfastly denying any involvement in the crimes while displaying an unwavering loyalty to Cath. Despite mounting evidence and accusations, Gwen never wavered from her stance, presenting a stark contrast to Cath's manipulative behavior.

The partnership between Cath and Gwen, though fraught with unanswered questions and conflicting accounts, stands out as a chilling example of how two individuals, intertwined in a web of deceit and manipulation, could orchestrate a series of heinous acts that shocked a community and baffled law enforcement. Their story serves as a haunting reminder of the complexities of human nature and the sinister potential lurking beneath seemingly ordinary facades.

Beatrice Yorker (1998) speaks in such a case of a 'leader' and a 'follower', or as the French term is 'folie à deux', where often it remains unclear who has what role. In the extensive Viennese murder-case in the next chapter, four nursing aides operate, in various combinations, killing one patient after another.

8.

The Lainz case

Waltraud Wagner, Irene Leidolf,
Stephanija Mayer, Maria Gruber, Austria, 1983

Oral Hygiene

Amidst the hushed corridors of a hospital ward in Austria, a trio of nursing aides cloak their sinister intentions under the guise of routine oral care. Dressed in their crisp blue-and-white uniforms, they move with calculated precision, their actions shrouded in secrecy.

In a chilling scene reminiscent of a noir thriller, they gather around the bedside of Herr Zeller, a frail figure lost in the shadows. With a whispered command, one of the assistants takes charge, wielding a jug of water and a spatula with deadly intent.

As the unsuspecting patient lies helpless, they perform their macabre ritual, manipulating his mouth with a cold efficiency. But this is no ordinary dental procedure; it's a calculated act of euthanasia veiled in the innocent guise of 'oral hygiene'.

With practiced ease, they silence their victim, the room falling eerily quiet save for the faint sound of stifled breaths. Then, as swiftly as they came, the women vanish into the darkness, leaving behind only the lifeless form of their latest victim.

This chilling tale of deception and death, unfolding over six long years, would later come to light as the notorious 'oral hygiene' murders, a grim

83

reminder of the darkness that lurks beneath the facade of medical care, where the line between mercy and murder blurs with chilling clarity.

Hospital Ward D

The morning of April 10, 1989, dawned with shocking headlines splashed across the pages of Vienna's newspapers *Mass Murder Uncovered in Lainz Hospital's Internal Medicine Department.* In a city known for its opulence and cultural heritage, the revelation sent shockwaves through the community, drawing comparisons to the atrocities of Nazi experimentation.

Nestled along the majestic Danube, the sprawling Lainz Hospital standing as a beacon of medical care, boasting eight pavilions that housed the city's most vulnerable. However, within the confines of Hospital Ward D, an insidious horror lurked beneath the facade of healing.

This ward, recently renovated but perpetually overcrowded, served as a grim haven for the city's elderly and infirm. Patients languished in crowded wards, their suffering compounded by the relentless bustle of hospital life.

The sinister truth came to light through the whispered confession of a nurse, shared over schnaps in a dimly lit café with her physician boyfriend. With trembling words, she revealed a chilling tale of betrayal and death: the clandestine administration of a lethal injection by a fellow nurse, resulting in the immediate demise of a patient. Yet, gripped by fear of repercussions as an immigrant and unwed mother, she chose the path of silence, burying her secret deep within the confines of her conscience.

Her revelation sparked a chain of events that would shake the foundation of Lainz Hospital. As her doctor boyfriend grappled with the weight of her confession, he sought counsel from his superior, an esteemed internist. But when their pleas for justice fell on deaf ears, they knew they had no choice but to take matters into their own hands.

With steely determination, they turned to the authorities, determined to unearth the truth behind the shadows of Hospital Ward D. A harrowing tale of deception and despair would be brought to light, revealing the chilling depths of human depravity lurking within the heart of Vienna's most esteemed hospital.

The Haunting Reality

Within the walls of Hospital Ward D, a chilling tale unfolds that would send shivers down the spine of even the bravest souls. Like a scene ripped from a spine-tingling horror film, this ward operates under the guise of medical care, but its reality is a nightmare for both patients and staff alike.

Chronic understaffing plagues the department, leaving overburdened nursing aides to tend to an overwhelming number of patients, upwards of forty each, without proper training or even a moment to attend to their own basic needs. The medical hierarchy is a tangled web of authority, with little more than orders exchanged between staff members.

In this chaotic environment, nursing aides take on tasks far beyond their qualifications, including administering medications and injections, while attempts to delegate these responsibilities to trained nurses are met with fierce resistance. Desperate for recognition, these assistants grasp at any opportunity to elevate their status amidst the chaos.

But the troubles don't end there. Supervision from management is virtually non-existent, leaving the department to spiral further into disarray. Meanwhile, whispers abound of scandalous affairs between the internist and two rival female departmental doctors, their tangled relationships casting a shadow over patient care.

Outside of working hours, the doctors are as elusive as ghosts, neglecting their duty to provide adequate pain relief for suffering patients.

Main Suspects

After the investigation begins, a dark and chilling saga unfolds, centered around the enigmatic figure of Waltraud Wagner. With the allure of an ordinary young woman, she effortlessly draws three others into her orbit, forming a quartet that would become infamous as the 'Angels of Death from Lainz'.

Yet, what sets this tale apart is its haunting subtlety. There are no flamboyant personas or overt signs of malice among them. These women defy the typical profile of female serial killers, lacking the usual markers of promiscuity or traumatic childhoods. Instead, they harbor a shared childhood dream of becoming nurses, just like Irene Becker from chapter 4, a passion that belies the sinister depths of their actions.

When an investigation into the rumors begins in February 1989, the detectives encounter a wall of silence, because according to the internist there is nothing wrong. But after staff was questioned, in addition to the 30-year-old main suspect Waltraud, 29-year-old Irene Leidolf, 48-year-old Stephanija Mayer and 26-year-old Maria Gruber were also taken into custody.

Waltraud

The truth slowly emerges, as Waltraud Wagner, the main suspect, confesses with chilling precision. Her admission of mercy killing 39 individuals sends shockwaves through the community, laying bare the depth of her actions.

Yet, in this intricate web of deceit, blame is not easily assigned. Waltraud implicates her accomplices, sparking a tangled web of accusations and counter-accusations. The internist, too, faces scrutiny for his failure to heed the warning signs, his excuses crumbling under the weight of scrutiny. Because, how could the most terrible things happen for six years and no one noticed? His excuse is that he had noticed that many patients died during Waltraud's shift. But during a renovation between 1987-1988, the subject was forgotten. The fact that people regularly died of natural causes also significantly delayed the discovery. The oral hygiene was not noticed because fluid can collect in the lungs even in terminal patients.

Are we dealing here with emergency workers acting out of force majeure, who worked under appalling conditions, far beyond their capabilities? Except for Reinhard B. from chapter 3, we have seen mean traits in the other perpetrators so far. Were they also present here, and especially at Waltraud? Cause amidst the shadows of unspeakable acts, she stands out. With the grace of a dancer and the resilience of a survivor, she emerges as a central figure in the harrowing tale that unfolds.

Born into a family of six daughters, Waltraud's journey begins against the backdrop of her grandmother's suffering, a haunting memory etched into her young mind as she witnesses the relentless agony eased only by morphine's merciful touch.

As she matures, Waltraud's path diverges from the conventional, abandoning her nursing studies at twenty to embrace a role as a nursing aide. Within the hospital's walls, she exudes warmth and compassion, a beacon of hope in a sea of suffering. Yet, beneath her cheerful facade lies a tumultuous inner world plagued by headaches and bouts of depression, struggles she navigates without the aid of medication.

Life's trials only intensify when her father's sudden departure shakes the foundation of her existence, leaving her to find solace in the unwavering support of her younger sister, a confidante unaware of the hidden depths within Waltraud's soul.

In the midst of this turmoil, Irene Leidolf emerges as a trusted companion, their bond forged in moments of shared laughter and quiet conversations over coffee. But beyond Irene, Waltraud's relationships with the other suspected nursing assistants remain shrouded in mystery, their ties veiled in the shadows of Hospital Ward D's secrets.

When confronted with the crimes that unravel the fabric of their reality, Waltraud's language betrays a peculiar nuance, a distinction between 'assistance in dying' and the stark reality of 'killings'.

Behind the cheerful demeanor of this young woman lies a chilling revelation: it was the most demanding and vexing patients, in Waltraud's perception, who met their demise. A retired teacher, known for his eloquence, allegedly escaped death only because Waltraud feared his potential betrayal if he survived her attempt on his life.

Irene

Then there's Irene Leidolf, slender and tall, with a younger sister as her only companion. Despite her intelligence, Irene's aspirations for a nursing career falter after failing her final exam. Nevertheless, she finds herself employed as a nursing aide on the ward, renowned for her sunny disposition and unwavering dedication. Her personal life, marred by tragedy and illness, adds layers of complexity to her character, from the heartbreak of a pregnancy, giving the baby up for adoption and a boyfriend's suicide to the agonizing experience of caring for her father as he succumbed to a malignant tumor.

Stephanija

And amidst this cast of characters stands Stephanija Mayer, the elder stateswoman of the group, her weary appearance belying a lifetime of hardships. Born in former Yugoslavia, her childhood is marked by turmoil, from witnessing partisan attacks to narrowly escaping drowning. Her memories are etched with visceral fear, making even the mention of 'oral hygiene' an unbearable reminder of past traumas.

Stephanija emerges as the standout intellect among the four women, her journey marked by twists and turns that mirror the complexities of her character. After completing four years of high school, she forgoes further academic pursuits to enter the workforce, eventually finding herself in a factory. A brief stint as a nanny follows before she embarks on a course to become a caregiver.

However, fate takes an unexpected turn when she marries a man consumed by jealousy and bitterness at the tender age of twenty. Their union leads to parenthood, but the marriage is short-lived, and Stephanija finds herself fleeing to Vienna, a city where she is a stranger and the language unfamiliar. Despite these challenges, she lands a job working with disabled children before her path ultimately leads her to Ward D.

Maria

Meanwhile, Maria Gruber, the fourth woman in this intricate tale, presents a stark contrast with her introverted nature and unassuming demeanor. Born into a household dominated by three sisters, Maria's upbringing is overshadowed by her father's role as the patriarch, a police officer tasked with maintaining order.

Completing high school and a year of vocational training, Maria embarks on a nursing career like her counterparts but finds herself at a crossroads, dropping out of the program and opting instead to work as a nursing assistant in a sanatorium. Her journey leads her to Hospital Ward D in 1983, where she quickly rises to the position of head nursing assistant, all while navigating the complexities of her personal life, including a pregnancy that prompts a temporary hiatus from work. Just like Irene and Stephanija, she cares for her sick father until he dies.

Degrading

In the shadows of Lainz Hospital's Ward D, a chilling tale unfolds as Waltraud weaves her sinister web, employing three distinct methods to extinguish the lives of her unsuspecting patients. Initially, she opts for potent doses of sedatives or insulin, but as time progresses, she increasingly turns to what she chillingly refers to (as we know) as 'oral hygiene'.

During a fateful night shift on Pentecost in 1987, Waltraud and Irene stumble upon a distressing scene: an elderly man sprawled on the floor beside his bed, an iron rod ominously nearby. Despite the patient's son filing a complaint, the cause of this unsettling incident remains shrouded in mystery, evading any definitive explanation.

Maria sheds light on Waltraud's macabre methods, revealing her preference for targeting patients already grappling with pulmonary edema. With a calculated hand, Waltraud administers not only water but also a cocktail of sleeping pills or additional medication down their throats, prolonging their suffering for hours, sometimes even a harrowing half-day, before their final breath.

In a courtroom charged with emotion, Waltraud's attempt to justify her actions as acts of compassion is met with a scathing rebuke from the prosecutor, who condemns her methods as nothing short of degrading. Yet, amidst the allegations and accusations, the evidence for her crimes remains frustratingly elusive.

Autopsies yield conflicting results, some hint at a drowning-like scenario, while others reveal traces of unauthorized sedatives. Nevertheless again, conclusive proof remains feeble. Even a colleague's account of witnessing Waltraud administer a non-prescribed injection provides little clarity on its contents.

As the trial unfolds, and under the weight of accusations from her peers, Waltraud finally succumbs to the pressure, confessing to the chilling reality that she is responsible for the deaths of nine patients. Yet, in the labyrinth of legal proceedings and fragmented evidence, the full extent of her crimes remains hauntingly obscured, leaving behind a chilling tale of deception, betrayal, and the harrowing consequences of misplaced trust.

In the courtroom, Irene recounts her unease with Waltraud's actions, admitting her habit of hastily exiting the sickroom whenever Waltraud embarked on her disturbing routines. Yet, a stark contradiction arises from a witness's testimony, alleging that Irene once unleashed a chilling warning upon a neighboring patient, declaring, 'If you keep nagging like this, you're next!' Tragically, the repercussions of that uttered threat would be realized the very next day, sealing the fate of the unfortunate patient.

Delving into the psyche of healthcare workers in emotionally charged settings, renowned psychiatrist Karl Heinz Beine sheds light on the pervasive use of dark humor as a coping mechanism amidst stress and suffering. However, as Beine astutely observes, healthcare serial killers take this seemingly innocuous behavior to sinister extremes.

Amidst the Chaos

As the trial unfolds, colleagues provide damning accounts of Stephanija's demeanor. Known for her sharp tongue and perpetual dissatisfaction, she becomes a focal point of scrutiny. Perhaps her own struggles, including managing high blood pressure with medication, contribute to her acerbic disposition. Stephanija, burdened by the relentless demands of the job, draws parallels between the pre-renovation Hospital Ward D and a harrowing refugee camp.

In a startling revelation, Stephanija eventually confesses to her involvement in the grisly 'oral hygiene' procedures, both in tandem with Waltraud and sometimes independently. However, amidst the fog of memory, she struggles to recall the frequency of her actions, leaving a lingering air of ambiguity and suspicion hanging over the courtroom.

Then Maria steps forward to share her side of the harrowing tale. Soon after joining the hospital staff, she overhears murmurs among colleagues about Waltraud administering fatal injections. Disturbed by the rumors, Maria chooses to ignore them, unable to fathom the possibility. Even when Waltraud herself introduces Maria to the concept of 'oral hygiene', Maria dismisses it as beyond belief.

Amidst the chaos, two deaths cast a shadow of suspicion, with accusations flying between Waltraud and Maria. Waltraud points the finger at Maria, alleging that she administered lethal doses of sedatives to both victims. In stark contrast, Maria insists she was a mere bystander, recounting a chilling encounter where Waltraud pressured her into injecting a painkiller into a suffering patient. Overwhelmed by the authority and unable to resist, Maria complies, unaware of the consequences until days later when the patient's life slips away. Faced with the grim reality of her unwitting involvement, Maria grapples with profound remorse, adamantly denying any involvement in the sinister 'oral hygiene' rituals. She estimates that 100 if not 200 patients may have fallen victim to these procedures.

The defense attorneys for all four women stand firm, highlighting the lack of concrete evidence in the courtroom. Despite the gravity of the accusations, doubts linger, shrouding the proceedings in a veil of uncertainty.

Parallels

What can we discern from the three notable resemblances among these four suspect women? Firstly, it's striking that three out of the four dedicatedly tended to a sick parent during their twenties and thirties. Waltraud witnessed her grandmother's illness firsthand, while Stephanija provided care for both of her parents until their passing. Irene, especially, bore the emotional weight of nursing her terminally ill father. Losing one or both parents at a young age profoundly impacted all four of them.

Secondly, the shared experience of failing to complete their nursing education led them to be relegated to the perceived inferior role of nursing aides, for the rest of their careers. This not only meant lower wages but also confined them to tasks they deemed unpleasant.

While their true motivations may never be fully unveiled, there could be an unconscious motive hidden within these parallels. Did their daily struggles with menial tasks under adverse working conditions exacerbate their frustrations? Or did the administration of pain relief take on a life of its own, escalating from bad to worse?

The Verdict

As the court's verdict echoes through the room, Waltraud Wagner crumples to her knees upon hearing the sentence: life imprisonment for fifteen murders and seventeen attempted murders. Tears stream down Irene Leidolf's face as she too receives a life sentence for five murders and two counts of complicity in murder. Stephanija Mayer remains stoic as the judge pronounces her sentence: twenty years for seven attempted murders and 8 to 24 counts of complicity in murder. Maria Gruber, unable to bear the weight of her sentence, covers her eyes with trembling hands as she learns she'll spend fifteen years behind bars for two attempted murders. Yet, her sentence is later reduced to twelve years on appeal, citing her young age at the time of the crimes and her inability to break free from Waltraud's influence. The internist, was dismissed from his position due to his late response to the rumors.

In 2008, when Waltraud Wagner and Irene Leidolf are released for good behavior, Austria reels with widespread shock. The revelation that Stephanija Mayer and Maria Gruber had been previously released, provided new identities, sends shivers down the nation's spine. The media coverage of this case not only reveals the dark depths of human depravity but also serves as a twisted inspiration for the perpetrator in the next chapter, mirroring the heinous acts of Frans H. from Chapter 1. Which makes her the second perpetrator who imitates crimes.

9.

Angel of compassion

Martha U., The Netherlands, 1995

Predicting

Because most perpetrators have malicious tendencies, the often-used motive of 'compassion' quickly becomes unbelievable. Only with Martha U. and the main character of chapter 17, Terri Rachals, there has never been such malice.

Born into a South Moluccan family in 1953, Martha's upbringing in the remote corners of the Netherlands was marked by hardship and resilience. Nestled amidst the sprawling landscapes of Ambonese refugee camps, she found solace in the simplicity of life, unaware of the sinister currents lurking beneath the surface.

At the tender age of 22, Martha embarked on a journey of service, joining the ranks of Vliethoven, a Christian psychogeriatric nursing home nestled in the heart of Delfzijl, a small town with an important port in the Northern Netherlands. Where her arrival was met with whispers of admiration, her commitment to the residents of Cedar ward unparalleled.

For 22 years, Martha's presence graced the halls of Vliethoven, her unwavering dedication a beacon of hope for those in need. From the darkest hours of the night to the brightest moments of the day, she stood as a pillar of strength, her compassion transcending the boundaries of duty.

But behind the facade of benevolence lay a darkness that few dared to acknowledge. As whispers of discontent echoed through the corridors of Vliethoven, Martha's personal life unraveled, her marriage crumbling beneath the weight of unspoken truths.

And then there was her son. Against her wishes, he slipped through her fingers, leaving behind a trail of heartache and regret.

As the years passed, Martha's once unshakeable faith wavered, the shadows of doubt creeping ever closer. And amidst the turmoil of her own making, she found herself teetering on the brink of despair, her angelic facade crumbling. And Martha U., once a pillar of dedication and compassion, finds herself thrust into a whirlwind of suspicion and uncertainty.

As the demands of her work escalate, Martha seeks solace within the confines of her profession, her home a mere shell of its former self without her trusted confidant by her side. Faced with resistance from her patients, Martha's frustration simmers beneath a facade of composure, a storm brewing within.

Yet, it was Martha's uncanny medical intuition that set her apart. Doctors marveled at her prognostications, particularly when she whispered chillingly accurate predictions about a patient's impending departure. Even in her personal life, Martha seemed to navigate effortlessly, her reputation as pure as the driven snow. In the close-knit community of her Moluccan Protestant church, she was regarded with reverence, her presence in the gospel group a testament to her unwavering faith. In the eyes of many, she was more than just a caregiver, she was a pillar of strength and a guiding light.

Yet, as the weight of her responsibilities grows heavier, she is forced to retreat, succumbing temporary to illness. But even in her absence, Martha's impeccable reputation remains untarnished, a testament to her unwavering dedication.

After working full time again, Martha's demeanor begins to shift, her once steadfast resolve wavering as she increasingly withdraws from meetings and consultations. Unbeknownst to her colleagues, Martha is slipping into the shadows, her actions cloaked in secrecy.

It is in the stifling heat of August 1995 that Vliethoven is plunged into turmoil, as the death of an 87-year-old patient on the Cedar ward raises suspicions. An investigation reveals a fatal overdose of insulin, prompting authorities to intervene. Yet, this is not an isolated incident; a previous death, shrouded in mystery three months prior, resurfaces, sending shockwaves through the facility.

As the truth slowly unravels, a pattern emerges: Martha U., the silent observer, present during each suspicious death.

Despair

In early September, Martha is arrested in her home, quickly confessing and admitting to being involved in the death of the 87-year-old man, acknowledging having killed at least four other patients by injecting them with a high dose of insulin. When Martha's lawyer visits her at the police station, he finds her in despair. How could this ever have happened? Only now does she realize that her actions were unacceptable. After five days of interrogation, Martha no longer eating, expresses a desire to die. As the judicial investigation progresses, there is suspicion that there may be a total of seven murders. The question that raises is, are we talking about premeditated murder or euthanasia gone awry?

By the end of September, Martha. Desperate is she banging her head against the wall, being prescribed antipsychotics and recanting some statements. At the urging of her lawyer, behavioral analysis is conducted.

Meanwhile, the revelations in the media stir up a lot of attention. Martha's arrest is a huge shock to many. Colleagues reacting with dismay. A well known newspaper in the North publishing messages of support. Martha is seen more as a hero than a cold-blooded murderer, many believing she committed the crimes following patient's wishes.

However, according to the chief prosecutor all evidence points towards murder, Martha, although suspected in nine cases, is charged with only four for evidential reasons. Just before the trial, the director of Vliethoven and one of the nursing home doctors break their silence. Martha did not kill out of compassion but out of frustration. All injected patients had strong, loving family ties, Martha herself lacked. Not wanting to tarnish their former employee's reputation, but these details would have come to light during the trial anyways.

Apart from the accusations, those two conveniently forget that the Angel of Death, as Martha is now called in the media, is one and the same as their own previously highly regarded staff member. Perhaps they should consider whether they might have overlooked warning signs.

Helping

In the crisp air of mid-December 1995, the hallowed halls of justice in the Netherlands bore witness to Martha U.'s long-awaited trial, a spectacle that drew a crowd of curious onlookers and fervent reporters. Among them coworkers, the grieving families of the victims, and a contingent of Martha's own kin, all awaiting the unfolding drama with bated breath.

As Martha's justice transport rolled into view, the scene erupted into a frenzy of flashing cameras and jostling reporters, each vying for the perfect shot of the woman at the center of it all. Only the firm intervention of police officers allowed the van to navigate through the throng and into the courthouse courtyard, where Martha's fate would soon be decided.

Inside the solemn confines of the courtroom, Martha cut a fragile figure against the backdrop of stern-faced judges adorned in their ceremonial robes. Her sleek hair was pulled back in a neat knot, and she wore a simple lilac sweater over dark trousers, a stark contrast to the gravity of the charges laid against her.

The allegations were damning: the suspect murdered completely helpless people and grossly abused the power she had in her position as a nurse. In 1994, she deliberately and premeditatedly injected a high dose of insulin to a man of 81 and a woman of 89, and in 1995 to a woman of 55 and a man of 87, after calm deliberation, after which the aforementioned patients died.

Crime Versus Mercy

The first victim, a fellow Moluccan, had reportedly been met with Martha's cryptic inquiry about his 'black suit', a cultural reference meaning that death is approaching.

In Martha's own words, spoken with a softness that belied the gravity of the moment, she revealed a heart torn between duty and compassion. Her actions, injecting the deadly dose, though ultimately fatal, were framed as acts of mercy, born from a wellspring of love and empathy for those in their final moments.

'Although Martha admitted during her initial confession to administering an overdose of insulin to the second victim', the prosecutor began, his voice cutting through the tension like a knife, 'she later retracted her statement, claiming a lapse of memory.'

Then came the haunting recollections of the last two victims, their lives cut short by Martha's alleged hand. 'The first victim', the prosecutor continued, 'a woman afflicted with the ravages of Huntington's disease, her body betraying her in the cruelest of ways. Unable to speak, her eyes beseeched Martha for relief, a silent plea for an end to her suffering'.

And the final victim, an octogenarian trapped in a failing body, yet his mind sharp as a blade.

According to Martha, he begged for help. Gasping for breath and feared losing his dignity. She also gave him an injection. When her colleague returned from her lunch break, Martha said that she would feed him herself, which he ate with relish, praying the Lord's Prayer together. When the first dose did not have the desired effect, she injects double the amount the next day. But, as the prosecutor points out, on the ward she had injected three of the four patients with insulin, letting the one in the worst condition live.

'And did you understand the consequences of your actions?' the judge's voice boomed, through the courtroom like thunder.

A nod from Martha, a fleeting acknowledgment of the darkness that consumed her soul.

Expert Witnesses

The court, unsatisfied with the meager revelations of the initial evaluation, turned to a psychologist and behavioral expert for a deeper dive into the depths of her psyche. Yet, amidst this new investigation, the echoes of the first assessment still lingered, casting a shadow of significance over the proceedings.

As revealed in the initial report, Martha's psyche was a labyrinth of afflictions, a portrait of turmoil painted with the brushstrokes of borderline personality disorder, a shattered self-image, masochism. But beneath the surface lay a darker truth: a thirst for power, a desire to commandeer the vulnerable, cloaked in the guise of benevolence. Martha's manipulative prowess knew no bounds, orchestrating a delicate dance of admission and denial to suit her whims, with a venomous bite awaiting those who dared challenge her authority.

In hindsight, Martha promotion to ward manager in 1990, despite her poor mental capacity, in combination with problems arising at home, proving a fatal combination.

But the past held more than just shadows; it whispered of warning signs ignored, of rage and defiance preceding the fatal injections. An 81-year-old man, his fury unleashed when Martha rebuffed his plea for solace, and a 55-year-old woman, her desperation manifesting in a violent act of defiance moments before Martha sealed her fate with a syringe.

In the intricate web of Martha's existence, these revelations were not merely details, they were threads woven into the fabric of her undoing, unraveling the layers of deception to expose the chilling truth beneath. As the courtroom witnessed the unraveling of Martha's psyche, a picture of chilling manipulation, power and the tragic consequences that followed emerged. In the chilling narrative of Martha's crimes, the second and final victim met their fate without a clash. It's a scene that speaks volumes, revealing a disturbing descent into masochism and self-destruction. The experts painting a picture of a mind teetering on the edge, rationalizing a fatal decision: if I administer the injection now, I'll be caught, and my

9. Angel of compassion

life will be forfeit. It's a chilling insight into the tangled web of Martha's psyche, where the lines between perpetrator and victim blur.

In the depths of Martha's mind, a neurotic character development unfolds, a compulsive need to play savior to the dependent, devoid of remorse. Remarkably, Martha stands firm in her resolve; given the chance, she would repeat her actions without hesitation. It's a stark revelation of a mind twisted by its own delusions, clinging to a warped perception of reality where the victims' wishes are twisted into justification for her heinous deeds.

The motive, as unveiled by the rapporteurs, lies in the tumultuous unraveling of Martha's personal life. Once a pillar of normalcy within her family, her world crumbled as her marriage faltered, and her authority was undermined by unforeseen defiance. From the ashes of her shattered existence emerged a torrent of suppressed aggression, fueling her descent into darkness. In the opinion of the court, which holds the suspect responsible for the nine murders she has confessed to, taking into account her reduced responsibility, she is sentenced to nine years in prison and compulsory psychiatric treatment.

Grateful

During the appeal Martha sat quietly, draped in a somber gray-black suit, her ebony hair pinned up in a bun with strands around her face. The air was thick with anticipation as the appeals process unfolded, casting a stark light on the tangled web of Martha's past and present.

As the expert witness took the stand, a former medical director of a psychiatric facility, the courtroom leaned in, eager to unravel the layers of Martha's psyche. His testimony painted a haunting portrait of a woman shaped by a childhood marred by neglect, abuse, and exploitation. Within the confines of her marriage, Martha faced a relentless onslaught of indignities, a constant barrage that wore down her resolve.

To navigate this minefield of trauma, she chose a profession as a care provider, which lends itself extremely well to a role in which she was not the underdog. But when she could no longer suppress her hurt in stressful situations, aggression escaped and those in need, paying the price. Martha completely lacking self-insight, still believing the victims are still posthumously grateful, as is often seen in rescue fantasies. She sees herself as the chosen one who had to save victims from their misery. Undergoing the prison sentence almost like a saint who passively sacrifices herself. Due to a significant risk of recurrence, it is recommended that she be treated therapeutically as soon as possible.

Reduced Sentence

During the appeal, the verdicts weren't solely weighed on Martha's shoulders. The findings of the Healthcare Inspection report cast a long shadow over Vliethoven, an institution where care should have been paramount, but where systemic failures marred its very foundation.

Picture Vliethoven: a sprawling complex housing 160 beds and a workforce of 300 souls, scattered across five wards. It was a place where, in 1995, residents weren't just housed; they were crammed four to a room, a far cry from the solitary or paired cells of Dutch prisons. And while the staff strove to create a semblance of comfort, darkness lurked in the cracks.

The whispers of discontent had started years earlier, in 1992, when the caregivers dared to speak out. They lamented a lack of camaraderie and respect from the physicians, echoing tales of favoritism and a culture of silence born from fear of reprisal. But grievances didn't stop there. The medical director, once seen as a beacon of authority, had lost the trust of his flock, while corners were cut and outdated practices persisted. Families of residents crying against the neglect they witnessed, while the staff grappled with mounting absences and an ever-increasing workload. Yet, their cries fell on deaf ears, as the management turned a blind eye to their pleas for change.

In the tapestry of tragedy that unfolded at Vliethoven, Martha's actions were but one thread, woven into the fabric of institutional neglect and apathy.

In the intricate dance between healthcare and oversight, Vliethoven emerged as a familiar stage for the Healthcare Inspectorate's scrutiny.

Martha's performance came under the microscope, revealing a troubling narrative. In 1994, amidst her prolonged absence due to illness, the first and only performance evaluation in over two decades was conducted. Martha's habitual avoidance of meetings remained unaddressed, as did her gradual withdrawal into herself. Opportunities to discuss weighty matters like euthanasia were missed, lost in the shuffle of institutional oversight.

In the courtroom drama, Martha's attorney weaves a compelling narrative, arguing that the Inspection report lays bare Vliethoven's shared culpability. With management neglecting their duty and leaving Martha to fend for herself, she descended into a dark abyss, ultimately resorting to destructive acts. But the Prosecutor General counters, asserting that organizational failure doesn't absolve Martha of her personal responsibility for the crimes.

As the verdict is delivered in Martha's absence during the appellate court proceedings, a hushed anticipation fills the room. The Court's decision is pronounced: four years in prison with compulsory psychiatric treatment, a reduced sentence. Even within the confines of prison walls, Martha's innate compassion shines through. In 1998, after serving two-thirds of her term, she is transferred to a mental health facility where her treatment journey begins.

10.

A kind of habit

Efren Saldivar, United States, 1989

Lack of Remorse

In the year 1989, a quiet unease settled upon the Glendale Adventist Medical Center in California, its corridors whispering with suspicion and fear. Little did the patients know, their trust in the healing hands of the medical staff would be betrayed by one of their own.

Efren Saldivar, a seemingly dedicated respiratory therapist, stood accused of a chilling series of crimes that would shake the community to its core. It wasn't until 1997 that the truth began to unravel, as whispers of unnatural deaths echoed through the halls of the medical center.

As the investigation unfolded, it became clear that Efren Saldivar was no guardian of life, but rather a predator lurking in the shadows of the hospital's sanctity. With each revelation, the weight of his crimes bore down heavily on the hearts of those left behind, their grief mingling with anger and disbelief.

In a courtroom fraught with tension, Efren Saldivar faced his accusers, his facade of innocence crumbling beneath the weight of damning evidence. Yet, even as the truth was laid bare, there was a chilling lack of remorse in his demeanor, a coldness that sent shivers down the spines of all who bore witness to his facade. 'Why' asks the judge did he became a respiratory therapist 'to help people?', Efren shakes his head. He just likes the uniform so much.

Despite his desperate attempts to evade justice, Efren Saldivar's reign of terror came to a decisive end as the gavel fell, sealing his fate with the finality of six life sentences plus fifteen years. But for the families of his victims, the wounds he inflicted would never fully heal, a reminder of the darkness that lurked within the heart of one who had sworn an oath to heal.

Child of Immigrants

In the rugged landscape of Brownville, Texas, amidst the dusty plains and scorching sun, a new life began in 1969. Efren emerged into the world, the son of hardworking Mexican immigrants who dared to dream of a better future for their family across the border.

Their journey fraught with challenges, but driven by hope and determination, they crossed into the land of opportunity, where the promise of superior medical care and the allure of American citizenship awaited their unborn child. With two-year-old Efren in tow, they made their way to the outskirts of Los Angeles, carving out a modest existence in a world pulsing with ambition and possibility.

Amidst the hustle and bustle of their new life, Efren's parents labored tirelessly to make ends meet. His father, gifted with skilled hands, embarked on a venture as a handyman, while his mother, a devout Jehovah's Witness, stitched together a livelihood by sewing clothes at home, her faith guiding every stitch.

Raised in the sheltered embrace of his family's beliefs, Efren and his younger brother found solace in the teachings of their mother, whose unwavering devotion to her faith permeated every aspect of their upbringing. Together, they embarked on Sunday missions, leaving behind the comforts of home to spread the word door-to-door, their hands laden with the weight of Watchtower magazines.

Despite the challenges of assimilation, the Saldivar children thrived, their grasp of English slowly solidifying as they navigated the unfamiliar terrain of American schools. Efren, a cherubic presence in his formative years, was deemed an average student, his teachers enamored with his sunny disposition, though they noted a certain naiveté born of his insular upbringing.

Significant

At the age of twelve, Efren spent a few weeks hospitalized with a complicated foot wound. The events left such a profound impression on him that he deemed this period the most significant in his life. He painstakingly detailed in an essay the procedure in which a doctor used a long needle to extract pus from the wound. Even as an adult, he vividly recalled the numbing sensation of the pain-relieving injection that dulled his skin. As puberty emerged, Efren began to undergo a transformation. He neglected his schoolwork and sought acceptance among older boys, only to find himself isolated when they failed to see value in him. Additionally, he failed his final exams. His interactions with girls also faltered; perhaps they deemed his 125-kilogram weight as simply too much. The repeated rejections fueled Efren's obsessive desire for women, culminating in the discovery of a hundred pornographic videos during a later search of his home. Efren's lack of initiative was evident, as he continued to reside with his parents until his arrest at the age of thirty-two. Despite being known as a helpful young man, he possessed a talent for deception. While he briefly took antidepressants, he eventually discontinued their use.

It's well-established that the upbringing of a serial killer is often characterized by absent parents and abuse. Numerous scholars highlight the impact of growing up in a dysfunctional family on the development of psychopathic or antisocial behavior. However, aside from potential taunting about his Mexican appearance as a child of non-white parents, Efren had a notably ordinary upbringing. Whether his crimes can be attributed to abnormal brain activity, as discussed in Chapter 3, remains unknown. However, a witness expert later testified that Efren suffers from an anxiety disorder.

Authority

In the tumultuous landscape of Efren's adolescence, a chance encounter at the age of sixteen sparked a revelation that would alter the course of his destiny forever. Working diligently as a store clerk in a supermarket, he witnessed the awe-inspiring authority exuded by ambulance personnel as they responded to a medical emergency. In that moment, amidst the hum of fluorescent lights and bustling aisles, Efren's vision of his future crystallized.

With unwavering determination, Efren pursued his dreams relentlessly. At seventeen, he defied the odds to obtain his high school diploma, a feat that laid the foundation for his journey into the world of healthcare. A year later, he emerged triumphant, graduating with honors from his training as a respiratory therapist. Clad in the distinguished attire reminiscent of a seasoned physician, Efren felt a surge of pride as he stepped into his newfound realm of responsibility.

His role as a respiratory therapist was more than just a job; it was a calling. Tasked with enhancing the lung function of patients battling respiratory ailments or tethered to ventilators, Efren's dedication knew no bounds. With precision and care, he meticulously calibrated inhalation medications based on the intricate nuances of each patient's oxygen levels, all while seamlessly assisting in life-saving resuscitation efforts.

Despite the challenges and uncertainties that littered his path, Efren remained steadfast in his pursuit of independence. For nearly a year, he navigated the maze of healthcare facilities, patiently awaiting an opportunity to claim his rightful place in the permanent night shift. For Efren, the night shift wasn't just a job; it symbolized autonomy and self-reliance in a world where he was determined to carve out his own destiny.

In the dawn of 1990, Efren's lifelong aspiration blossomed into reality as he clinched a coveted position at the Glendale Adventist Medical Centre.

But Efren's devotion extended beyond the confines of his newfound role; for three additional years, he also toiled through endless night shifts at another hospital, driven by a singular mission to save enough to gift his mother a car.

Efren's dedication was unwavering, and his diligence bore fruit as he garnered an impressive depth of knowledge in the realm of medicine. His expertise soon soared to remarkable heights, positioning him as a peer among physicians and shattering any remnants of doubt surrounding his capabilities.

As time unfolded, Efren seamlessly transitioned into the role of overseeing the permanent night shift at the Glendale Adventist Medical Centre, assuming the mantle of authority and independence. His solitary companion in the dimly lit halls was scarcely seen, their duties carefully divided at the onset of each shift, tending to patients scattered across different wards. For eight illustrious years, Efren thrived within the institution's walls, his performance standing unblemished despite whispers of speculation lingering in the air.

Anonymous Tip

The ominous whispers about Efren, swirling long before his eventual arrest, had given rise to a chilling moniker among his colleagues at the hospital 'Magic Syringe'. It was a nickname steeped in dark irony, as patients tended to meet untimely ends shortly after receiving injections from Efren. A group of respiratory therapists, perhaps sensing something awry, once delved into Efren's locker in jest, only to stumble upon a cache of opiates and syringes. Despite their unsettling discovery, they chose to remain silent, opting to brush off their concerns.

However, one therapist, grappling with a nagging sense of guilt, couldn't shake off the troubling suspicions. Summoning the courage to voice his concerns, he confided in the department head. Yet, amidst a tangled web of office politics and personal animosities, his warnings fell on deaf ears. Instead of heeding the whistleblower's plea for investigation, the department head, swayed by preconceived biases, chose to silence the accuser, suspending him as a gesture of loyalty to Efren.

But fate has a way of revealing its secrets in the most unexpected of ways. During a casual evening at a local pub, one of Efren's colleagues, fueled by liquid courage, inadvertently spilled a damning secret to an individual with a dubious past. Sensing an opportunity for extortion, the individual anonymously tipped off the hospital authorities, alleging that a respiratory therapist was orchestrating premature endings for unsuspecting patients.

In a tragic twist of fate, the hospital administration, blinded by misplaced loyalty or perhaps a desire to avoid scandal, chose not to escalate the matter to law enforcement. Unbeknownst to them, their inaction set in motion a series of events that would haunt them for years to come.

As another year dawned, a second anonymous call pierced through the veil of complacency, prompting the administration to finally sound the alarm. With a third anonymous call following in quick succession, the urgency of the situation became starkly apparent, time was running out, and lives hung in the balance.

Shush

In the heart of California, a dedicated team of investigators delves into the intricate web surrounding Efren Saldivar, their suspect in a chilling case. A journey beginning with a close examination of those who orbited Efren's world. Unraveling the threads of his relationships reveals a disturbing pattern.

One of Efren's former colleagues steps into the spotlight, offering insights into the enigmatic figure. Describing Efren as outwardly normal, she recalls unsettling conversations where he confessed a desire to ease the suffering of others by hastening their departure from this world. An eerie hush descends as she recounts a haunting scene: Efren, with a finger pressed to his lips, urging silence as a nurse prepared to intervene in a patient's final moments.

Yet, the shadows hold darker secrets still. Another witness emerges, shedding light on Efren's troubling actions. With a heavy heart, this witness reveals Efren's admission of an accidental injection of a potent muscle relaxant into a patient's veins, an action far beyond the scope of his duties.

As the investigation deepens, attention turns to a colleague whose loose lips reveal damning truths. In a courtroom confession offered in exchange for immunity, she lays bare the depths of Efren's depravity. Yes, she had supplied the lethal substance to him, desperately trying to intervene as he wielded it with deadly intent. Yet, in a chilling twist, the specifics elude her memory, the patient's name, the aftermath of the overdose.

Despite her immunity, the toll is severe. Her career lies in ruins, stripped of her professional standing for her role in facilitating death and concealing the truth. In the haunting echo of Efren's actions, lives are forever altered, and the specter of his crimes casts a long, dark shadow over all involved.

Spotlight

As the cloud of suspicion looms over Efren, measures are swiftly taken to keep him at a distance from the hospital corridors, his shifts rearranged to ensure a safe distance. When the detectives finally corner him for questioning, Efren, as if driven by an urgent need to unburden his soul, spills his secrets without hesitation. However, after 48 grueling hours of interrogation, the police are compelled to release him, lacking the tangible evidence needed to keep him behind bars. With tearful farewells, Efren expresses heartfelt gratitude to his interrogators, leaving his attorney to later dismiss his confessions as coerced and unreliable.

In the wake of grave suspicions, the hospital swiftly cuts ties with the respiratory therapist, severing their once-close association. In a final gesture of contrition, he reaches out to his former employers, offering apologies for the tumult he has caused.

As we have noticed this Health Care Serial Killer thrives in the spotlight. Like Irene Becker of chapter 4, he likes the publicity and grants a riveting television interview, vehemently refuting any connection to the sinister events and brazenly declaring his confessions to be nothing but fabrications. His demeanor, both on television and the sterile courtroom, paints a portrait of a man teetering on the edge of madness. Dying his hair and retreating to the solitude of a remote vacation home, only to find the seclusion unbearable.

Returning to the rhythms of ordinary life, Efren takes up employment at a car rental agency by day and becomes a nighttime pizza deliveryman. He even dabbles in a brief stint as a nighttime dispatcher until his face graces the front pages of newspapers, heralding a lawsuit from the bereaved families of patients whose lives were cut short under suspicious circumstances.

By the scorching summer of 2000, Efren vanishes into thin air, leaving behind a swirling vortex of unanswered questions, marking yet another chapter in the enigmatic saga of Efren Saldivar.

Bewilderment

As the investigation unfolds, it gradually reveals a staggering truth: over the course of the eight years Efren spent at the hospital, more than a thousand patients met their demise either just before or during his presence. With an average of 250 workdays per year, this equates to an alarming rate of involvement in a death every other day, a statistic that leaves detectives scratching their heads in bewilderment. Where does one even begin in the face of such overwhelming numbers? Yet, the crux of the matter, as always, lies in assembling the elusive pieces of evidence.

A total of twenty bodies are exhumed from their resting places. Enter Brian Andresen, the relentless forensic toxicologist, whose unwavering determination leads to a breakthrough: a groundbreaking test capable of detecting traces of the muscle relaxant in the tissue of the deceased. Finally, after three arduous years since the initial involvement of law enforcement, the crucial evidence emerges, leading to the long-awaited moment when the suspect is finally apprehended, his hands shackled in the unforgiving embrace of justice.

Efren's response is surprisingly subdued. Before even stepping foot into the police car, he boldly expresses his preference for the ultimate punishment: the death penalty. Yet, as the officers escort him into the station and ceremoniously remove his restraints, his demeanor shifts, offering reassurances in a strangely self-effacing manner. 'Fear not', he quips, 'for I am such a coward that escape is beyond my realm of bravery'. Yet beneath the veneer of nonchalance, there lingers a hint of curiosity, as he jests about potential surveillance, playfully tapping on the microphone and offering a mischievous 'test, test' to those listening in. And when his rights are read aloud, a formality he could easily rebuff, he simply waves them aside with a casual disregard, as if the weight of his actions were but a fleeting concern.

Routine

At first, Efren adamantly denies any wrongdoing, but soon his story unravels into a tapestry of contradictions. His confessions, initially coherent, become disjointed as he struggles to maintain a grasp on reality. In a moment of erratic behavior, he fixates on the mirror before him, questioning its transparency like a character in a detective novel, all while sipping lemonade through a straw. His memory of the number of victims wavers, oscillating between ten, ninety, or even two hundred, with a confession to losing count after the initial sixty. Yet, amidst this confusion, he recalls a temporary decrease in his killing spree after his colleagues intruded into his private space.

During interrogation, Efren offers a medley of perplexing motives. He claims a cowardly aversion to suicide led him to seek the death penalty by committing a second murder. He fancies himself an 'Angel of Death', convinced of his victims' readiness to depart this world. Amidst these delusions, he reveals a xenophobic belief in safeguarding the hospital from non-contributing immigrants, oblivious to his own immigrant roots. His resentment toward prolonging the lives of terminally ill patients adds another layer to his twisted rationale.

As recounted by the tireless lead detectives, Efren's modus operandi emerges. He meticulously selects victims from the patient list, guided by his skewed criteria and a disdain for those he deems unworthy of life. His actions, unnoticed by his colleagues, evolve into a chilling routine.

A psychiatric expert paints a portrait of Efren's psyche, attributing his crimes to paranoia and a desire for revenge against a world that perceived him as weak. His lack of remorse, a hallmark of his psychopathic nature, further illustrates the depths of his depravity.

The judge's verdict holds Efren accountable for his deeds, despite his attempts to fabricate motives during questioning. When pressed for remorse, Efren's cavalier response underscores the callousness of his actions.

In Efren's own words to the court, 'Your Honor, initially, there was a twinge of conscience, but eventually, killing became as trivial as stealing a pack of gum. You do it without a second thought, and afterward, it simply fades from memory'.

11.

Godmother

Beverley Allitt, England, 1991

Diverged

In the quiet village of Gorby Glen nestled in the heart of the English Midlands, a sinister figure lurked in the shadows of innocence. Beverley Allitt, born in 1968 as the second child in a modest household, possessed an unsettling aura that set her apart from her peers from an early age.

From the onset, it was evident that Beverley's path diverged sharply from the norm. Alienated from her classmates during her formative years, she sought solace in solitary moments, her presence a haunting specter against the backdrop of the schoolyard fence.

But beneath her façade of determination lay a labyrinth of deceit and manipulation. Her relationships, marred by betrayal and deception, served as mere pawns in her sinister game of control. Her lack of academic prowess served as a testament to her tumultuous journey, as she stumbled through the trials of high school, her dreams of nursing teetering on the brink of oblivion. Yet, against all odds, Beverley's perseverance bore fruit as she finally grasped her diploma at the age of twenty-one, a harbinger of the horrors yet to unfold within the confines of the pediatric ward.

Self-Harm

In the eerie corridors of Grantham & Kesteven General Hospital, nestled close to her hometown, the enigmatic tale of nurse-in-training Beverley Allitt unfolds with sinister overtones. Her journey through the ranks of medical education is fraught with a disturbing pattern of self-inflicted harm and baffling illnesses that raise unsettling questions about her fitness for the noble profession of caregiving.

Born in 1968 amidst the serene backdrop of Gorby Glen, Beverley's early years hinted at a troubled soul. A solitary figure during school breaks, she harbored dark secrets beneath her withdrawn facade. Troubling episodes of self-harm, including injuries inflicted with a hammer and deliberate encounters with glass shards, cast a shadow over her already tumultuous existence.

As adolescence beckoned, Beverley's descent into darkness spiraled further. Neglecting academic pursuits, she wandered into the abyss of delinquency, seeking solace in the company of a rebellious clique. Her nights were shrouded in intoxication, a haze that clouded her senses and led her astray from the path of virtue.

But amidst the chaos of her troubled mind, a flicker of ambition emerged, a desire to heal, to nurture, to don the mantle of a nurse, particularly in the realm of pediatric care. Yet, Beverley's journey toward this noble calling was marred by deceit and manipulation, a disturbing pattern that would later unravel with chilling consequences.

During her tenure at the hospital, Beverley's behavior bordered on the macabre. Repeated visits to the Emergency Department for self-inflicted injuries, feigned ailments, and a disturbing penchant for inserting urinary catheters until they broke off and required surgical removal painted a chilling portrait of a disturbed mind lurking beneath her nursing uniform.

Despite her questionable track record and a trail of red flags, Beverley's ascent through the ranks of nursing was inexplicably unhindered. Her presence on the pediatric ward, where she was initially rejected but later granted a temporary appointment, sent shivers down the spines of those who crossed her path.

In the shadowy world of healthcare, where trust and compassion are paramount, Beverley Allitt's story serves as a cautionary tale, a chilling reminder that darkness can lurk behind the most seemingly benign facades, waiting to unleash its malevolent wrath upon the unsuspecting souls who dare to tread its treacherous path.

Suspicion

In the corridors of the hospital where Beverley Allitt had recently embarked on her nursing career, whispers of concern began to circulate after a string of unsettling incidents unfolded under her watchful eye.

A mere six days into her tenure, chaos erupted when a seven-week-old infant, struggling with pneumonia, suffered a sudden respiratory arrest. Beverley's swift action averted tragedy, as she sounded the alarm and led the successful resuscitation efforts. Yet, the joy of this fleeting victory was soon overshadowed by tragedy when, just days later, the same infant succumbed to another respiratory crisis, this time with fatal consequences.

In a chillingly short span of time, another child met a similar fate, falling victim to an inexplicable cardiac arrest under Beverley's care. As suspicions mounted, a grim pattern emerged, raising eyebrows among both staff and parents alike.

The atmosphere within the hospital became fraught with tension as colleagues, while outwardly commending Beverley's apparent diligence, exchanged knowing glances laden with unspoken doubts. Yet, amidst the shadows of suspicion, Beverley remained an enigmatic figure, her actions veiled in a cloak of uncertainty.

As the casualties mounted and the hospital corridors whispered with rumors, a sense of unease settled over the once bustling wards. With each passing day, the weight of suspicion grew heavier, casting a pall over the hospital's once bright halls. And in the midst of it all, Beverley Allitt lingered, a silent specter haunting the hospital's darkest recesses.

In the span of just three days, Beverley's brazen actions sent shockwaves through the hospital's corridors as she dared to strike again, this time in the presence of over a dozen staff members, tending to a fifteen-month-old toddler. With less than five weeks under her belt on the ward, she seemed undeterred by the risk. Yet, what transpired next was nothing short of chilling.

Beyond Comprehension

A five-month-old infant, seemingly healthy, suddenly lapsed into unconsciousness within the week. Beverley's astute suggestion of a potential diabetic coma proved eerily accurate, a diagnosis confirmed upon examination. The incident repeated itself not once, but twice more, leaving a haunting pattern in its wake.

In a cruel twist of fate, two children, unsuspecting and innocent, were thrust into the grip of sudden cardiac arrests within days of each other. Once again, it was Beverley who raised the alarm, though her demeanor during resuscitation efforts was noted to be strangely detached, her gaze distant and unfocused.

As the number of resuscitations skyrocketed, suspicions among Beverley's colleagues grew, with thirteen such incidents in just a month, a staggering contrast to the hospital's historical average. Yet, the inconceivable notion that a trusted member of their team could be intentionally putting patients in harm's way remained beyond comprehension, delaying the urgent response that could have saved lives.

In the eerie calm that followed, a chilling realization dawned upon the hospital staff: April's arrival heralded a sinister resurgence of inexplicable tragedies, leaving them grappling with the haunting question of who, or what, was truly behind the unfolding horrors.

Twins

In the haunting halls of Ward 4, the arrival of a four-month-old pair of identical twin girls, daughters of a friend of Beverley, marked another tragic sequence of events. With just a week between their admissions, the first twin's passing shortly after discharge shook the hospital to its core. Concerned, the second twin was admitted for observation, a decision that would reveal chilling truths about the sinister presence lurking within.

Under Beverley's watchful eye, the second twin's condition took a perilous turn, requiring resuscitation three times during Beverley's shift. The desperation of the parents, enveloped in grief, met with Beverley's seemingly comforting embrace, as she was credited with saving the life of their surviving daughter. Yet, beneath the facade of gratitude lay a chilling lack of remorse, as Beverley's acceptance of the godmother role for the remaining twin betrayed an unsettling indifference to the tragedy that had unfolded.

In the wake of the twin's deaths, forensic examinations uncovered a harrowing truth, traces of insulin overdose and another unknown substance tainted their bloodstreams, casting a dark shadow over Beverley's presence on the ward.

As the days unfolded, the specter of tragedy loomed ever closer. A six-year-old boy's life slipped away after an antibiotic injection, carelessly left unattended in Beverley's presence. A four-week-old infant faced three near-death emergencies, while a seven-week-old baby suffered lasting brain damage under Beverley's watchful eye.

In the chilling silence of Ward 4, a two-month-old infant became the final victim. As life ebbed away, Beverley stood motionless, her presence a looming specter of death. The discovery of poison during the autopsy only deepened the shroud of suspicion surrounding Beverley's inexplicable actions, leaving Ward 4 haunted by the sinister legacy of the Angel of Death who walked among them.

Fine Line Between

More than a week passed since the last tragic loss before authorities were called in to unravel the disturbing mystery haunting Ward 4. But what they uncovered was beyond staggering, a web of missing medical records, lab results, and crucial reports, all pointing to one name: Beverley.

In a startling turn of events, the search for evidence led detectives to Beverley's doorstep, where the damning missing files were shockingly found in her possession. With this revelation, Beverley's role in the unsettling chain of events could no longer be denied, leading to her suspension from duty.

Desperate to avoid the glare of media scrutiny, Beverley sought refuge with a trusting friend, who, blinded by loyalty, refused to believe the allegations against her. Even as suspicion mounted, this friend offered her shelter, conveniently allowing Beverley to lend a helping hand in the care of her children, unaware of the danger that lurked. Even when her youngest child becomes unwell, she refuses to believe that Beverley could be blamed. Only afterwards can it be determined that Beverley added glucose-lowering tablets to the boy's soft drink. But Beverley's charm wasn't limited to just one individual. The parents of the twin girls, whose lives she was credited with saving, couldn't fathom the possibility that their guardian angel could be anything but innocent. In a bid to clear her name, they enlisted the help of a private detective, clinging to the hope of vindication.

Despite the mounting evidence against her, Beverley's supporters remained steadfast in their belief, viewing her as a savior rather than a suspect. And though Ward 4 may have returned to a semblance of calm, the shadow of doubt cast over Beverley's actions lingered, a chilling reminder of the fine line between savior and perpetrator.

Showcasing

When the nurse was apprehended a week following the last resuscitation, she exuded an unsettling calmness, as if the event were a mere formality rather than a pivotal moment in her life. With an air of nonchalance, she submitted to the authorities, seemingly unfazed by the gravity of the situation unfolding around her. Initially, she adamantly denied any involvement in the incidents that had rocked the hospital's pediatric ward.

It wasn't until her conviction that the facade of innocence shattered, revealing the true extent of her actions. Confessions emerged, detailing how she had administered doses of five different medications to nine children initially, with a further admission of four more. Shockingly, in the case of the final victim, she confessed to a chilling act of manipulation, placing a towel over the child's face with the sinister intention of later showcasing her resuscitation skills. With an unsettling serenity, Beverley claimed that three of the victims had met their demise purely by accident.

Yet, behind the veneer of composure during her initial interrogation lurked signs of a deteriorating mental state. During her pretrial detention, she succumbed to the throes of anorexia nervosa and inflicted self-harm, a stark contrast to her outwardly composed demeanor. This troubling revelation painted a grim picture of her inner turmoil, juxtaposed against the cavalier tone of letters penned to friends and the parents of the twin girls. In these missives, she callously joked about the inconvenience of postponing her vacation plans due to the trial and anticipated using her eventual compensation to bolster her wardrobe upon release.

Adding another layer of distress to her troubled history, it was unearthed that Beverley had previously worked several night shifts at a nursing home, where one resident narrowly escaped a diabetic hypoglycemic episode, casting a chilling shadow over her past actions.

Münchhausen

In the courtroom, the prosecutor paints a chilling tableau: eleven harrowing attempts at murder, four tragic deaths, and countless acts of violence against innocent children.

But amidst the somber proceedings, a perplexing dichotomy emerges. Despite the weight of the evidence, a faction of the pediatric ward staff staunchly defends their former colleague, Beverley. They speak of her as a devoted caregiver, seemingly attentive to the needs of her young charges. Yet, upon closer scrutiny, their descriptions paint a picture of a nurse whose interactions were clinical and devoid of the compassion expected in such a role. There's a discomforting undercurrent as they recall Beverley's meticulousness, an unsettling intensity that left them uneasy.

As the case unfolds, experts delve into the labyrinthine corridors of Beverley's mind, revealing a young woman ensnared in a web of insecurity and profound psychological turmoil. Driven by an insatiable craving for attention and validation, she resorts to acts of self-harm and manipulation, a tumultuous existence bereft of remorse or empathy.

Beverley Allitt's story takes a dark turn as she becomes the poster child for Münchhausen syndrome. This revelation casts a shadow over her actions, reminiscent of Münchhausen by proxy syndrome, where caregivers harm their charges to garner sympathy and attention. In Beverley's twisted narrative, she inflicts pain upon helpless children under her care, seeking validation through her role in their resuscitation efforts.

Life Sentence?

In the aftermath of the trial, a contentious report titled *The Clothier Report* or *The Allitt Inquiry* ignites a fiery debate. Advocacy groups square off against safety agencies in a battle over the employment of former psychiatric patients in caregiving roles, sparking broader conversations about mental health and accountability within the medical community.

In 1993, Beverley faced the harsh judgment of the court, receiving thirteen consecutive life sentences for the murder of four children, attempted murder of three others, and deliberate infliction of harm on six innocent kiddies. Just three months post-conviction, Beverley found herself back under medical care for self-inflicted stab wounds and a disturbing attempt to ingest glass shards, revealing the depths of her inner turmoil.

During her incarceration, Beverley's life took a curious turn when she found companionship in an unlikely place, a relationship blossomed with a female fellow inmate, a robust pyromaniac, offering her a modicum of solace in her grim circumstances.

But the legal saga didn't end there. In 2007, as the prospect of release loomed on the horizon under England's policies for life-sentenced individuals, Beverley found herself devoid of supporters advocating for her freedom. At a subsequent hearing, opponents challenged the initial diagnosis of Münchhausen syndrome, pointing out the shortcomings of the expert witness in the original trial. They argued that Beverley's actions, rife with psychopathic and sadistic undertones, warranted a different judgment, a declaration of mental incompetence. However, the die had been cast, and Beverley's fate sealed.

The plot thickened as it emerged that Beverley's time behind bars was spent predominantly in a psychiatric hospital due to her disruptive behavior. This raised troubling questions about the integrity of her punishment. Was she effectively evading the consequences of her actions in a facility where discipline was lax, and autonomy over her life held sway? The debate raged on, shrouding Beverley's future in uncertainty.

In a decision handed down by the High Court of Justice, a path toward treatment within the prison system was mandated for Beverley, with a glimpse of hope for the future. It was decreed that, should she demonstrate rehabilitation and earn society's trust once more, she could potentially be eligible for release after serving a minimum of thirty years behind bars, accounting for time served during her pretrial detention.

12.

Recommended

Genene Jones, United States, 1981

Certificate

We have seen hospital officials apply ostrich policy before, but the staff of San Antonio Medical Centre in Texas really buries its head deep in the sand. During the first 24 months of her employment, Genene Jones works in the Emergency Department, but because she presents herself almost as often as a patient in the waiting room as she assists the doctor, she is transferred to the pediatric intensive care unit.

Yet, even in this specialized setting, Jones's sinister intentions became apparent. A disturbing pattern emerged as children under her care inexplicably perished, sending shockwaves through the medical staff.

Colleagues, disturbed by the escalating death toll, voiced their concerns to the head nurse, only to have their fears dismissed. Meanwhile, Jones's lethal incompetence reached its zenith when she nearly administered a fatal dose of anticoagulant to an unsuspecting patient, attributing the near-tragedy to a mere 'miscalculation'.

As the body count continued to rise under her watchful eye, it became abundantly clear that Jones's tenure at the medical center was marked by a reign of terror rather than a commitment to healing.

In a belated acknowledgment of her egregious actions, Jones was ultimately relieved of her duties, receiving the following certificate:

Nurse Genene Jones, born on July 13, 1950, was employed by the San Antonio Medical Centre from October 1978 to March 1982. Her departure is completely unrelated to the quality of her work. Throughout her employment, she was known as a loyal, reliable staff member possessing valuable knowledge and experience. She was an asset to our hospital, and we can therefore highly recommend her employment.

Ill Luck

Genene is lovingly taken into their family by affluent parents as their third adopted child shortly after her birth in the southern Texan city of San Antonio. Within a year, the trio is joined by another boy. All the children attend the Catholic elementary school and taking turns having piano lessons on Wednesday afternoons. A listening mother after school and playing by the pool. Father owns a nightclub and a couple of restaurants. But despite how peaceful this picture may seem, Genene felt like the black sheep in the family. Clashing with her mother, and as much as her father is kind to her, she feels disgusted by the girl she sees in the mirror.

At the age of ten, the first shock comes: father having cracked a safe is taken to the police station. Although he confesses, the charge is ultimately dropped for unknown reasons.

Once in high school, the second blow occurs: her younger brother dies after a homemade bomb exploding in his face. Although Genene deeply affected by the accident, she is back in the classroom the afternoon after the funeral, where her classmates surround her with interest. Loving the attention might have been the core of her later addiction to being (here we go again…) in the spotlight.

The once idyllic family life lay in ruins, irreparably damaged beyond recognition. And yet, the storm had not yet passed, for while Genene thrived academically, her father was dealt a devastating blow: cancer. At the tender age of eighteen, she bid farewell to him as he succumbed to the relentless disease.

Genene's world crumbled beneath her feet, leaving her adrift in a sea of grief. Her mother, unable to bear the weight of loss, sought solace in the bottle. But Genene sought a different path, a way to escape the suffocating despair that threatened to engulf her.

At eighteen, she concocted a tale of pregnancy, weaving a narrative that led to an ill-fated marriage with a former classmate. Despite her mother's initial resistance, the charade persisted, leading to a union shrouded in deception. Settling into the confines of her mother's estate, Genene played the role of dutiful wife while her husband toiled as a mechanic before venturing into the navy.

In the absence of her husband, Genene sought comfort in the arms of another, a fleeting respite from the turmoil that plagued her existence. When her husband learned of her infidelity, he chose to turn a blind eye, perhaps weighed down by his own burdens.

As fate would have it, tragedy struck once more when her older brother succumbed to the same merciless disease that had claimed their father. Yet, amidst the wreckage of loss, Genene refused to surrender to despair. Instead, she charted a new course, embarking on a quest to become a beacon of beauty.

Her dreams of becoming a beautician were dashed by a cruel twist of fate, as she developed an allergy to the very products she hoped to wield. Undeterred, she forged ahead, giving birth to a son before bravely seeking divorce.

Undaunted by the challenges that beset her, pursuing a career in nursing with unwavering determination, excelling in her studies. Just newly graduated as a practical nurse at the age of 27 when in 1977 her second child, a daughter, is born.

Guardian Angel

At twenty-eight, her name already carried whispers of trouble through the halls of San Antonio Medical Centre. Genene's past was tainted with swift departures from two previous hospitals, where she had been ousted after just eight and two months respectively. Her transgressions were stark: dispensing medication without authority and hurling insults at a specialist.

But despite her tarnished reputation, Genene found herself welcomed into the fold of San Antonio's emergency department. Here, she danced a dangerous tango of flirtation with the attending physicians, while her children remained nestled in the care of her mother, moving to her own apartment.

As the year turned to 1981, Genene's path took a fateful turn. A transfer landed her in the pediatric intensive care unit, where she assumed the mantle of the night shift. Despite her role as a practical nurse, she conducted herself as if she were the matron herself, holding court with parents and dismissing doctors' directives with a wave of her hand.

Yet, beneath her facade of authority lurked a dark truth. Eight times, she administered the wrong medications, each time risking the fragile lives under her care. And once, in a brazen display of recklessness, she stumbled onto the unit inebriated, accompanied by a companion who dared to tamper with vital equipment. Her colleagues recoiled in horror, their whispered concerns echoing through the sterile halls. But in the face of a crippling staff shortage, their voices fell upon deaf ears. The head nurse, blinded by necessity, shielded Genene from the consequences of her actions, clinging to her as a lifeline in the storm of overwork and understaffing.

Obsessed

In the shadowed corridors of healthcare, a sinister obsession festers, gripping the hearts of several notorious figures, Genene Jones among them. They are afflicted with a morbid fascination known as thanatophilia, a twisted preoccupation with all things deathly. But it's not just the departed they fixate upon; it's their own mortality too, a theme we'll revisit with the chilling tale of Charles Cullen in Chapter 21.

Amidst the chaos of Genene's arrest, the harrowing testimonies of parents echo hauntingly. One recalls her macabre gesture of holding a lifeless infant up to the heavens, as if offering it as a sacrificial lamb. Another recounts the chilling sight of Genene, eyes ablaze with an otherworldly fervor, frozen in place as their own child teetered on the brink of eternity. And when death claimed the innocent soul, the nurse's reaction was nothing short of chilling, tears streaming, she positioned herself beside the lifeless form, a mournful sentinel in the dimly lit room, though her connection to the child was scant at best.

The eerie trance enveloping Genene begs for an explanation. In Chapter 4, delving into Irene Becker's story, and Chapter 6, unfolding Michaela Giersberg's tale, we witnessed the haunting phenomenon where caregivers find echoes of their own anguish in the suffering of others, where, as it were, merges. When the floodgates of their own hidden agony crack open, they're trapped in a hypnotic dream state.

My research, detailed in my book *Engelen des Doods* (2007), revealed that this altered mental state afflicted a significant quarter of perpetrators, a chilling revelation of the darkness lurking within the souls of those sworn to heal.

Teddy Bear

In the somber echoes of tragedy, the voices of grieving parents reveal chilling encounters with Genene Jones, shrouded in the enigma of her actions:

With trembling hearts, parents recall the haunting sight of Genene, cradling their lifeless infants in her arms, her mournful wails mingling with the shadows of the nursery. Despite the customary transport of the deceased on a gurney, Genene insisted on carrying the tiny forms herself to the mortuary, a gesture both unsettling and intimate.

Yet, it was in the solemn sanctuary of the graveyard that the true depths of Genene's obsession with death unfurled. Unbeknownst to grieving parents, who sought solace beside their child's grave, they stumbled upon Genene, a spectral figure kneeling in the twilight. Rocking back and forth, whispering the names of the departed, tears mingling with the earth, as if communing with souls long departed. The sudden intrusion shattered her reverie, and like a ghost vanishing into the night, she retreated into the shadows, leaving behind only unanswered questions and a stolen memento of grief. In the hushed aftermath of these encounters, the specter of Genene Jones looms ever larger, her presence a dark enigma in the lives of those touched by tragedy. Especially when they noticed that she had also taken a teddy bear from the grave.

Pitfall

In the depths of the pediatric intensive care unit, a chilling pattern emerged between May 1981 and January 1982, shrouded in inexplicable tragedy. Children, though far from the edge of life, succumbed to mysterious hemorrhages, seizing bodies, and cardiac arrests, leaving doctors grasping at shadows in search of answers.

In one harrowing instance, a six-month-old baby suffered an epileptic seizure followed by also a cardiac arrest in Genene's presence. Despite successful resuscitation efforts, the infant bled from every orifice, a sight that sent shivers through the staff. Though they managed to stabilize the bleeding temporarily until Genene's subsequent late shift. When the baby displayed the same symptoms once more, it was too late to save them, the cause of death remaining elusive.

As grief gripped the heart of a devastated father, a cruel twist of fate awaited him. While doctors rushed him to the urgent care ward, Genene callously placed the lifeless child upon its sibling's lap, only to snatch it away and flee to the cold embrace of the mortuary, leaving the family bewildered and bereft. Her actions defied comprehension until an autopsy revealed a lethal dose of anticoagulant in the infant's system.

In the wake of yet another inexplicable death, Genene's audacious actions reached new heights of incomprehensibility. As physicians stood in stunned silence, she approached the bedside of the fallen child and traced a watery cross upon its brow, echoing the same gesture upon her own, a baffling ritual that left witnesses grasping for meaning in the depths of the unknown.

Prevailing Disbelief

By the dawn of October 1981, after eight agonizing resuscitations, colleagues could no longer ignore the whispers of suspicion that swirled around Genene's presence. With mounting concern, they sought solace and answers from the physicians, clinging to the faint hope of unraveling the shadowy web that ensnared their unit in a veil of despair.

Once again, Genene Jones finds herself under the protective wing of favoritism, as the chief clinician hails her as the shining star of the unit. Any whisper of her potential involvement in the unsettling occurrences is swiftly dismissed as paranoia by a dissenting doctor, who soon finds himself sidelined and eventually ousted from his position. This lamentable pattern exposes the prevailing disbelief that any member of the staff could be capable of such heinous deeds, obstructing the early detection of the unfolding tragedy due to a veil of ignorance.

Despite the mounting concerns among the unit's staff, a consensus emerges that action must be taken, leading to the implementation of stringent protocols: every administration of anticoagulants now requires double verification by a second staff member, with one vigilant doctor even committing to sleeping on-site, poised to catch any sinister activity. Yet, despite these precautions, the grim specter of tragedy persists, shrouded in a cloak of mystery.

Genene, forever beset by nebulous ailments, voluntarily seeks admission for observation, yet her maladies remain unclassified. However, as the holiday season of 1981 approaches and Genene resumes her duties in her crisply starched uniform, the death toll rises once more, claiming the lives of six innocent children under inexplicable circumstances. Even in the face of evidence suggesting anticoagulant overdose in two of the victims, the elusive nurse remains elusive, evading detection with uncanny ease.

It isn't until a vigilant doctor catches Genene consulting a medical manual on the clandestine administration of injections that alarm bells finally ring, prompting a long-overdue intervention from hospital management. In early 1982, a distinguished professor of anesthesiology from Toronto Hospital for Sick Children arrives, armed with insights from a similar ordeal in 1980, where 43 deceased patients in the cardiology unit were discovered to have been administered excessive doses of heart stimulants, the source of which remained an enduring enigma.

Private Clinic

Amidst the whispers of hushed corridors and the lingering scent of tragedy, a clandestine maneuver takes shape to rid themselves of Genene without igniting the flames of public scrutiny. A decree emerges from the upper echelons of management: henceforth, only registered nurses, not practical nurses, shall tread the corridors of the intensive care unit.

With the aforementioned certificate in hand, Genene is quickly led out the door, leaving a trail of unanswered questions behind.

Yet, fate has other plans in store, as Dr. Kathleen Holland, a pediatrician embroiled in the tangled web of hospital politics, sees through the smokescreen of institutional maneuvering. She views Genene's dismissal through the lens of the hospital's entrenched machismo, a perspective that leads her to extend a lifeline to the ousted nurse. Ignoring the cautionary whispers of her peers, Dr. Holland invites Genene to join her in the establishment of a new venture: a private medical practice nestled in the serene confines of Kerrville, a haven located a hundred kilometers northwest of the chaos they leave behind.

On August 1, 1982, amidst the sweltering heat of summer, Genene steps through the doors of Dr. Holland's private clinic, her new title of pediatric clinician a badge of honor, meaning a level of expertise that far exceeds her qualifications. As the tendrils of fate entwine their paths, the shadowy allure of the private clinic beckons, promising sanctuary amidst the tumultuous storms of professional upheaval.

For Kathleen, medicine transcends mere profession; it's a sacred calling etched into the very core of her being. Within the walls of her private practice, she forges connections that defy conventional doctor-patient boundaries. Personally reaching out to parents to schedule appointments, she invites them to address her by her first name, fostering an atmosphere of familiarity and trust. With heartfelt dedication, she ensures that anxious parents are kept informed of their child's progress, her voice sometimes faltering with emotion as she relays updates over the phone.

Friends

Also, the relationship between Genene and Kathleen transcends the typical confines of employer and employee, veering instead into the realm of deep friendship. This blurred distinction clouds Kathleen's perception of the practical nurse, tilting the balance of power in Genene's favor. Their bond goes beyond professional duties, with Genene extending a welcoming hand to Kathleen, offering her temporary refuge in her Kerrville abode amidst ongoing renovations. In this symbiotic arrangement, Genene finds the supportive sister figure she's longed for, fostering an environment where after-hours conversations over cigarettes at the kitchen table become a cherished ritual, delving into topics ranging from fashion to life's twists and turns.

Adding to this intimate setting is the presence of the nanny, whose own baby becomes a fixture in Genene's household. In a moment of crisis, when the nanny's daughter falls gravely ill and requires urgent medical attention, Genene seamlessly assumes the role of a concerned grandmother, navigating hospital corridors with a blend of maternal instinct and steadfast support, seamlessly integrating herself into their lives with a bond forged in trust and mutual reliance.

Wake-Up

In the tranquil facade of the private clinic, a tempest of dread stirs. Eight young souls, innocently seeking treatment, are suddenly seized by respiratory arrest, echoing the haunting echoes of past tragedies in the pediatric intensive care unit. Urgent measures are taken, the whir of helicopter blades slicing through the air as all eight children are whisked away to the nearest hospital. Amidst the chaos, seven lives are salvaged, but the heart-wrenching toll claims one innocent victim. A fourteen-month-old cherub, once merely battling a slight sniffle, now lies still, her young life extinguished by a sequence of events shrouded in uncertainty.

A mother's anguished cries echo through the corridors as she recounts how her child received two injections from Genene mere moments before the onset of the harrowing seizures. Genene's demeanor, as she delivers the grim news to the parents, is chillingly composed, a facade of calm amidst the storm, while beads of sweat betray the turmoil within.

En route to the hospital, amidst the roar of the helicopter engines, a vigilant nurse witnesses a clandestine act: Genene administering another injection to the child, a prelude to the tragic final heartbeat.

In the aftermath, Kathleen, the stalwart guardian of the clinic, is confronted with a disturbing revelation. A vial of muscle relaxant, its rubber stopper punctured, is discovered, a silent witness to clandestine machinations. Kathleen's disbelief swells as she grapples with the realization that she never ordered nor sanctioned the use of such medication, casting a shadow of suspicion upon her once-trusted colleague.

Before she can unravel the web of deceit, Kathleen is thrust into another turmoil. Genene lies sprawled on the clinic floor, intoxicated and confessing to an overdose of antidepressants. The urgent rush to the hospital unfolds before Kathleen's eyes, a grim reminder of the fragile balance between life and death that hangs over her clinic. As uncertainty looms like a gathering storm, Kathleen fears for the very survival of the sanctuary she had painstakingly built.

Escape

Meanwhile, the executives at the San Antonio Medical Center, under the guidance of the Canadian professor, have been far from idle. The alarming spike in mortality rates cannot be dissociated from the presence of the departed nursing aide, prompting the intervention of law enforcement.

But as the net tightens around the elusive suspect, she slips through the cracks, evading accountability with a supposed suicide attempt that tests the resolve of Kathleen, the steadfast guardian of the clinic. With her children in tow, the suspect flees, vanishing into the horizon two hundred kilometers away.

However, the truth is a relentless pursuer, and soon, lurid headlines in tabloids cast the suspect in a damning light, linking Genene to a string of inexplicable child deaths while painting her as a deviant lesbian. Enraged by the scandalous portrayal, the suspect hastily enters into a marriage with a nineteen-year-old boy, a desperate bid to deflect the mounting scrutiny. But the deception is short-lived, as the law closes in with the swift precision of justice. Handcuffs replace wedding bands as the suspect's escape plan unravels in a moment of reckoning.

As detectives descend upon Kathleen's private clinic, her worst fears materialize in the form of damning evidence linking the suspect to the harrowing events. The once unassailable reputation of Kathleen crumbles under the weight of suspicion, her professional integrity tarnished by association.

Colleague physicians, once allies, now shun her, citing her alleged lapse in judgment in employing personnel of questionable character. Patient referrals dwindle to a trickle, and with the nearest hospital withdrawing its support, Kathleen is left with no recourse but to close the doors of her clinic, a sanctuary now tainted by betrayal.

Amidst the wreckage of her shattered dreams, Kathleen finds herself standing alone, abandoned even by her spouse, as she grapples with the aftershocks of the tumultuous downfall orchestrated by her former protégé.

Pride

With tears streaming down her face, Genene is led between officers towards the waiting police van, her demeanor a mix of sorrow and defiance. Yet, once seated at the interrogation table, a remarkable shift occurs. Suddenly composed, she eagerly engages with investigators, brushing aside her attorney's counsel to remain silent. Her words flow freely, a torrent of denial and defiance that belies her vulnerable facade. In a bold move, Genene addresses the media in a defiant press conference, vehemently refuting all accusations against her.

Behind bars, Genene's thirst for attention knows no bounds. In a chilling display of bravado, she seeks details of her fellow inmates' crimes, only to boast proudly of her own heinous deeds when the conversation turns to her.

Her hunger for infamy manifests in various elaborate schemes, from concocting fake death threats to feigning illnesses and even a phantom pregnancy. When her adoptive mother initiates proceedings to gain custody of her grandchildren, Genene sends her threatening letters. Her young husband divorces her.

While judicial departments focus on Genene, she faces charges in two separate courts in Texas. In Kerr County, she stands accused of the murder of the fourteen-month-old girl from the private clinic, while in San Antonio, the charges, despite extensive investigations, are limited to a single count of attempted murder and 27 suspected homicides. Throughout the trials, Genene remains an enigmatic figure, sitting stoically in the courtroom, her indifference to the gravity of her crimes a chilling testament to her unyielding pride.

Revelation

In the realm of healthcare serial killers, proof is thin as usual, and Genene Jones's case is no exception. Statistical analysis paints a grim picture: a child under her watch in the intensive care unit was twenty-five times more likely to succumb to a fatal cardiac arrest than under the care of another staff member. Yet, the threads of evidence are frayed, with crucial laboratory findings mysteriously vanishing into thin air, and the passage of time rendering exhumed bodies too decomposed for meaningful examination. Only in the tragic tales of a fourteen-month-old from a private clinic and a boy drained of life at the San Antonio Medical Center do traces of a lethal overdose emerge.

Delving into Genene's psyche, psychiatrists search for answers, but find no solace in declaring her mentally incompetent. Their quest for motive leads them down a labyrinth of perplexing conditions, from Münchhaussen by proxy syndrome to a hero complex, wherein Genene seemingly orchestrated perilous scenarios to play the savior, a twisted heroine snatching children from the clutches of death.

However, amidst the chaos, a bombshell revelation emerges from the shadows, shedding light on a potential motive that had remained hidden during her tenure under Kathleen's employ.

A nurse from the pediatric ward at the nearby hospital recounts a chilling exchange with Genene, wherein she inquired about the absence of an intensive care unit. When informed of the low volume of critical cases, Genene's response hinted at a deeper, more sinister agenda that sends shockwaves through the investigation. In the midst of this crisis, Genene offered a seemingly simple solution, asserting confidently, 'Those patients are out there, you just have to find them'. She went as far as suggesting that a future intensive care unit for children could be effectively managed by practical nurses alone.

Yet, as the legal proceedings unfolded, Genene's defense faltered, her attorney grasping for straws, merely suggesting that his client may have been overly dedicated to her work.

In a courtroom in Kerr County, the gavel fell with a resounding finality as Genene was sentenced to 99 years behind bars for the murder of the fourteen-month-old girl who tragically perished in the helicopter, effectively shattering any notion of Sudden Infant Death Syndrome as the cause of death. Meanwhile, in San Antonio, in addition to her Kerr County conviction, she will receive an additional sixty years on top of her Kerr County conviction for the attempted murder of the bled-out boy with an overdose of a decoagulant.

13.

Interplay of circumstances

Michaela Roeder, Germany, 1985

Favorite

Most European serial killers in healthcare have been caught in Germany, where this story takes place. Shortly after the publication of Karl Heinz Beine's book *Sehen, Hören, Schweigen. Patiëntentötungen und aktive Sterbehilfe* in 1998, as was already mentioned in the introduction, several major cases came to light. Whether this is because Germany is the largest European country or because attention to the subject led to perpetrators being caught earlier, remains a matter of speculation. In his research, Beine shows, among other things, a relationship between poor working conditions and the likelihood of someone turning to murder. A similar relationship seems to exist in the case of Michaela Roeder.

In 1978, newly qualified nurse Michaela begins her specialist training in anesthesia and intensive care at St. Petrus Hospital in Wuppertal, a city in the middle of the Ruhr area, northeast of Cologne. At first glance she appears to be a spontaneous, open-hearted young woman, working in an intensive care unit that is run in a strict, hierarchical manner by a female ward physician who tolerates no dissent. Besides a poor relationship between the doctors themselves and between doctors and nurses. Especially the latter feel abandoned to their fate.

In the tumultuous year of 1980, a formidable figure emerged within the surgical department's ranks, casting a shadow of authority and ambition. This new chief clinician, whose arrival heralded a surge in surgical procedures and an expansion of the intensive care unit, commanded respect from colleagues and subordinates alike.

Yet, within this realm of heightened activity and professional rivalry, a power struggle ensued between the chief and the ward physician, igniting a battle for control over patient care. As tensions flared, the ward physician found her influence waning, eclipsed by the chief's domineering presence.

Amidst this backdrop of internal strife, one individual stood out as an exception to the escalating tensions, Michaela. Having completed her specialized training, Michaela forged an unlikely alliance with the ward physician, earning herself a rapid ascent up the career ladder. However, this newfound favor came at a price, as rumors swirled about the nature of their relationship, casting a shadow of doubt over Michaela's integrity.

Isolated and burdened by the weight of her elevated position, Michaela struggled to maintain her professional facade. Overworked and overstressed, she succumbed to lapses in judgment, neglecting basic medical protocols and dismissing the needs of her patients with callous indifference.

But it was the revelation of the ward physician's personal struggles, her battle with alcoholism, that ultimately shattered Michaela's fragile equilibrium. Witnessing her mentor stumble through patient rounds in a haze of inebriation, Michaela's world spiraled into chaos, culminating in a catastrophic breakdown that would forever alter the course of her career.

Toilet Attendant

In the bustling city of Wuppertal, Michaela Roeder enters the world amidst the hopes and dreams of her young mother, just nineteen at the time. But from her first breaths, an unseen tension permeates the air between mother and child. Expecting a cherubic bundle of joy, Michaela's constant regurgitation disrupts her mother's carefully laid plans for motherhood, throwing her into disarray. Diagnosed later as pyloric stenosis, a swelling of the muscle between the stomach and the intestines, causing severe vomiting, setting the stage for Michaela's tumultuous journey. As she grows, defying societal norms by eschewing dresses for the rough and tumble of boys' games, her mother's hopes for a compliant daughter fade into oblivion.

Discord becomes a constant companion in the Roeder household as Michaela's unconventional preferences clash with her mother's expectations. While her father attempts to inject levity into the strained atmosphere, his efforts fall short against the weight of unresolved tension.

In the shadow of a troubled childhood, Michaela's path is set on a collision course with fate, where innocence is shattered and secrets lie in wait.

One day, Michaela overhears her mother confiding in the neighbor, 'My daughter's birth has ruined my entire life'. And when the girl doesn't excel beyond the average student in high school, her mother threatens, she'll end up as nothing more than a toilet attendant.

As the shadows of adolescence deepen, Michaela finds herself at odds with the expectations laid upon her. Threatened by her mother's ominous words should she fail to excel academically, Michaela's spirit remains undeterred. Despite her struggles in the classroom, she becomes the class clown, her laughter a shield against the weight of disappointment.

But life's twists and turns spare no one, not even the most innocent of souls. A brother's arrival brings both joy and envy, as Michaela watches her mother's affection lavished upon the newborn, while she remains an outsider in her own home.

Expulsion from school at fifteen marks a turning point, a crossroads where Michaela's path diverges from the conventional. It's only through tending to a disabled child that she earns a fleeting glimpse of her mother's approval, a rare moment of validation in a sea of uncertainty.

As the years pass, Michaela's journey leads her to the austere halls of St. Petrus Hospital, where she begins her training as a nurse. Despite her practical skills, she struggles to excel in theory. Yet amidst the academic challenges, she finds solace in the guidance of a childless teacher, unaware of the darkness of her alcoholic addiction. During one of her visits, Michaela just manages to stop her from jumping off the balcony.

Betrayed

At the tender age of nineteen, romance beckons to Michaela like a siren's call, promising love and affection. But fate deals her a cruel hand when she discovers her crush is already engaged, a harsh reality, followed by being raped by her driving instructor. Yet, amid the wreckage of shattered dreams, a glimmer of hope emerges as she qualified for her nursing degree, paving the way for a specialized training in anesthesia and intensive care.

In the midst of these professional milestones, a new chief clinician takes charge, and Michaela, buoyed by her rapport with the ward physician, excels in her specialization. With her own place to call home, her once-strained relationship with her mother finds solace in the pride of her daughter's achievements.

However, love's embrace turns sour at twenty-five when Michaela's heart is torn asunder by a man who hides a marriage beneath his charming facade. Shocked and betrayed, she severs ties with him, making up a tale of his untimely demise to mask the pain of her shattered dreams. Though the world may believe her fabrication, the truth remains buried beneath layers of deception and heartache.

With the specter of betrayal looming large, Michaela retreats from the realm of intimacy, leaving behind the whispers of a rumored affair with the female ward physician. Alone yet resilient, she navigates the tumultuous waters of love and loss, her spirit unbroken despite the scars that mark her journey.

Why?

September 17, 1985. As Wuppertal's residents savor the last warm days of summer, a 68-year-old man is wheeled into the intensive care unit after surgery. Michaela, an experienced nurse with a calm, confident air, makes a decision that will alter the course of the day, and the patient's life. She'll spare him further suffering. In doing so, she conveniently overlooks the crucial fact that agreeing to surgery is a clear expression of the will to live. And without hesitation, preparing a syringe and administering a fatal dose of blood pressure medication, his condition rapidly deteriorates. But Michaela is nothing if not methodical. Knowing her colleagues will call a doctor if they find him in such a state. Moving quickly, she follows up with another drug, ensuring his life ends quietly and without interference.

Six days later, a new patient arrives, a 70-year-old man, also post-surgery, unable to speak, only communicating through hand gestures and nods. Just hours earlier, a nurse confirmed the man felt well. That's why it's jarring when Michaela claims he's in severe pain and needs an injection.

Her colleague listens as she opens four ampoules in quick succession. Through a crack in the door, he sees her taking the patient's hand and administer the injection. Unease builds in his chest. Checking on the man a short while later, he finds his blood pressure critically low and alarmed, he insists they call a doctor.

'Why bother?' Michaela says, her tone icy. 'He's going to die anyway.'

Upon the doctor's arrival, he orders a plasma infusion to stabilize the man. But Michaela isn't done. 'Let it run in slowly,' she instructs, a curious directive given the urgency of the situation, cause plasma is supposed to be infused quickly to restore blood pressure.

The patient's heart monitor flatlines briefly, only to show a weak rhythm moments later. Michaela, clearly annoyed, mutters, 'Oh great, he's acting up again.' Sending her colleague to answer a phone call and once alone preparing another syringe. This time, her injection is final. The heart monitor flatlines, this time staying that way.

Later, Michaela will say to her colleague with unsettling calm: 'See! I know when the end is inevitable.' Leaving him shaken, but doubt clouds his mind. Did he really see what he thought he saw?

By morning, consumed with guilt, he confides in a trusted colleague and together they decide to watch Michaela more closely, clinging to the hope it was all a mistake. After all, how do you confront your superior with the chilling question: 'What exactly was in that syringe?'

Her Own Request

A little over a month later, a 79-year-old woman with a dire prognosis is admitted to the ICU. Michaela, convinced the woman is on the brink of a long and painful decline, decides to intervene. With practiced ease, she administers a hefty dose of blood pressure medication, followed quickly by another drug. The patient takes one final, shuddering breath and slips away.

Later that same day, another patient, a 67-year-old man on the mend, becomes her next target. Michaela delivers a lethal injection, and when his condition takes a sharp turn, the team scrambles to save him. During the chaotic resuscitation, the doctor calls for sodium bicarbonate. Instead of following the order, Michaela prepares a syringe containing yet another overdose of the same drug that started the crisis. Which, unaware of the deadly swap, the doctor administers, resulting in the patient's death.

Another month passes. On December 6, 1985, an 84-year-old woman is set to leave the ICU for a general ward, her recovery progressing well. But after reporting chest pain, her transfer is postponed, and she remains under observation. The day-shift nurse hands over her care to Michaela for the evening.

'She won't make it past midnight,' Michaela declares, her voice eerily matter-of-fact.

Later, Michaela would claim that during her first check that evening, the patient insisted she no longer wished to stay in the intensive care unit, a statement no one else could corroborate.

Without hesitation, Michaela administers an overdose of blood pressure medication, followed by the woman's nosedive vitals. Michaela, watching the numbers drop, remarks to a colleague with a sly grin: 'Her blood pressure is crashing.' Whereupon the alarmed nurse urges her to call a doctor, Michaela brushing him off: 'Why bother? She doesn't stand a chance anyways,' Michaela returning to the bedside and delivering a second, fatal dose.

Within minutes, the patient takes her last breath. After preparing the body for the morgue, Michaela logs the incident in her evening report with the chilling words 'transferred to the morgue at her own request.'

This time, the two nurses who have been quietly observing Michaela decide they can't remain silent any longer, confronting the attending physician, sharing their belief that Michaela is behind the unusual string of deaths in the unit.

However, their concerns are met with scorn. 'What's this really about?' the doctor asks, eyes narrowing. 'Are you perhaps after her job? Or did she turn you down?' Defeated and demoralized, the nurses retreat. Their warnings, like those before, fall on deaf ears. And Michaela, shielded by a mix of disbelief and indifference, continues her deadly routine unchecked.

Football Match

The saga unfolded with a sinister rhythm, each chapter darker than the last, as Michaela's actions plunged the hospital into a gripping tale of betrayal and tragedy.

Twice more, Michaela wielded her syringe like a weapon, handing over unsuspecting doctors a deadly dose that sealed the fate of their patients. Yet, despite the mounting evidence, the whistleblowers found themselves mired in a twisted web of disbelief and suspicion.

One of the courageous whistleblowers, driven by a relentless pursuit of truth, clandestinely retained vials of blood from one of the victims. Seeking validation for his suspicions, he sought the assistance of the laboratory under the guise of a sick pet, only to be confronted with a chilling revelation: the blood profile matched that of a creature already long deceased.

Nearly a month later, the somber echo of tragedy returned with devastating force. A 58-year-old woman, having undergone her second operation, found herself slipping away under Michaela's watchful gaze. As the ominous words escaped Michaela's lips, foretelling the woman's untimely demise before the kickoff of the Italy-Germany football match, the whistleblowers recoiled in horror.

Before leaving for the day, they meticulously counted the remaining vials of the blood pressure-lowering medication in the medicine cabinet, a precautionary measure to validate their suspicions. Driven by an unwavering commitment to justice, one of the whistleblowers, after a restless night's sleep, placed a direct call to the chief clinician to voice his concerns. Following deliberation, the chief confirmed the unfortunate passing of the patient at 2:00 p.m. Startled by the revelation, the nurse implored the chief to conduct a count of the remaining vials. The grim discovery of seven missing vials prompted the chief clinician to take swift and decisive action, immediately suspending Michaela, on grounds of suspected involvement in the untimely demise of several patients.

Despite their relentless pursuit of truth and their pivotal role in uncovering Michaela's nefarious deeds, the whistleblowers found themselves consigned to the shadows of obscurity, denied the courtesy of acknowledgment or gratitude for their vigilance, even in the face of overwhelming evidence implicating the culpable nurse.

Flashing Cameras

In the aftermath of Michaela's expulsion from the medical fraternity, a whirlwind of events catapults her into the spotlight of notoriety. With the permission of the now-involved police commissioner, she embarks on a two-week ski trip, seeking solace amidst the pristine slopes. Little does she know, upon her return, her sanctuary will be shattered.

Stepping through the threshold of her home, she is met with a scene of chaos, a raid has taken place, and her prized possession, her diary, is missing. Before she can process the situation, the heavy hand of the law intervenes, and she finds herself under arrest.

In a frenzy of emotion, Michaela's facade crumbles. Anger turns to despair as she lashes out, cursing her fate. But amidst the chaos, a moment of clarity emerges, and she collapses into tears, the weight of her actions finally catching up to her.

At the police station, amid the harsh fluorescent lights and sterile walls, Michaela's resolve wavers. With trembling hands and a heavy heart, she confesses to the unspeakable crimes that have haunted her every waking moment. Relief washes over her as she unburdens her soul, but the consequences of her actions are only just beginning to unfold.

Outside the confines of the interrogation room, a frenzy of media vultures descends upon the hospital, hungry for the latest scoop. Camera flashes illuminate the once-quiet corridors, transforming them into a stage for the sensational drama unfolding within.

Amidst the chaos, whispers of scandal and sensation echo through the halls. Sensational headlines paint a vivid picture of a forbidden romance between the suspect and the ward physician, weaving a tangled web of intrigue and deceit.

In the midst of this media storm, the whistleblowers find themselves thrust into the spotlight, offered a hefty sum for an exclusive interview. But true to their principles, they decline the offer, steadfast in their commitment to integrity and justice.

As the dust settles and the headlines fade, the tragic tale of Michaela Roeder serves as a cautionary reminder of the darkness that lurks beneath the surface, even in the most unsuspecting of places.

House of Cards

During her long pre-trial detention, Michaela is subjected to psychological and psychiatric observation for eight months, which leads to the following conclusion. As a child, the suspect felt rejected by her mother, which led her, in search of recognition, to first adore her teacher and later the female ward doctor. But when she could no longer deny the instability and alcoholism of her idols, her world collapsed like a house of cards and she found herself alone, both privately and professionally. Due to this conflictual situation, her feelings got the better of her and she developed omnipotence fantasies in the belief that she was chosen to prevent unnecessary suffering of patients. She is declared fully accountable.

In the dimly lit courtroom of Wuppertal, the stage was set for a trial that would capture the attention of a nation. Three years had passed since Michaela's arrest, yet the echoes of her alleged crimes reverberated through the halls of justice.

As she entered the courtroom, a flurry of camera flashes illuminated her path, turning her arrival into a spectacle fit for the silver screen. But amidst the chaos and clamor, Michaela stood defiant, her demeanor anything but that of a woman accused of orchestrating the deaths of 23 patients. With an air of confidence that bordered on audacity, Michaela, the accused, exuded a charm that seemed incongruous with the gravity of the charges against her. Her demeanor, reminiscent of a triumphant athlete basking in the glow of victory, betrayed no hint of remorse or guilt.

Guided by her attorney's counsel, Michaela turned to face the throng of reporters, her smile radiant as she posed for the flashing cameras. In that moment, she appeared more like a celebrity embracing the adoration of her fans than a defendant facing the specter of justice.

But as the commotion reached a fever pitch, the presiding judge intervened, his stern voice cutting through the chaos. 'Pack up your equipment. This is no entertainment', he declared, his words a sobering reminder of the gravity of the proceedings unfolding before them.

In the courtroom of Wuppertal, where justice hung in the balance, Michaela's trial would be a spectacle like no other, captivating the nation and leaving an indelible mark on the annals of criminal history.

Dual Responsibility

The courtroom became a battleground, the stage for a legal duel that would span 48 grueling days. Tensions ran high as the prosecution clashed vehemently with the defense, each side fiercely advocating its stance. The defense, unyielding in its strategy, pointed fingers at the ward physician, arguing that she bore a share of responsibility for the tragedy that unfolded. Meanwhile, the prosecution countered with a relentless barrage of accusations, contending that Michaela's intellect, with an IQ of 112, rendered her fully cognizant of the consequences of her actions.

As the trial drew to a close, Michaela seized the opportunity to address the court. Gone was the facade of confidence and bravado, replaced instead by a poignant confession. In a voice tinged with regret and sorrow, she uttered words that resonated throughout the courtroom, 'Today, I stand before you, bewildered by the events that transpired. When I acted, I believed I was fulfilling the wishes of the patients. Now, I see things differently. I deeply regret my actions and seek forgiveness'.

In the aftermath, the judge made a ruling that resonated with a sense of somber reflection. Michaela was found guilty on several counts, including manslaughter and attempted murder. But the departure from conventional sentencing recognized the complex interplay of circumstances and personality traits that led to her actions. And, in contrast to Martha U.'s sentence from chapter 9, it addresses Michaela's motive of compassion; she therefore receives a relatively light prison sentence of eleven years. Emphasizing she was not a callous killer, but rather a troubled individual who became entangled in a web of circumstances beyond her control. Because research has shown that both labor relations and medical care in intensive care must have been catastrophic, he also holds the hospital and the department doctor partly responsible.

As Michaela embarked on a new chapter of her life post-incarceration, she chose, like the nurse's aides of chapter 8, to fade into obscurity, adopting a new identity and seeking redemption through reintegration into society. Meanwhile, journalist Christiane Gibiec delved into the depths of the case, chronicling the intricacies of Michaela's story in her book, *Tatort Krankenhaus, Der Fall Michaela Roeder* (1990), shedding light on the complexities of human nature and the frailty of the human psyche in the face of overwhelming adversity.

14.

The infertile choir singer

Wolfgang Lange, Germany, 1990

Astor

In the year 1990, according to the ticking hands of time, a peculiar scene unfolded in the quaint German town of Gütersloh, nestled snugly southwest of the Teutoburg Forest. Picture this: a stout, somewhat weathered man, his countenance marked by the faint traces of a receding hairline and a modest goatee, strolls along the cobblestone streets, accompanied by his loyal canine companion. Now, had Astor, the faithful hound, possessed the uncanny ability to decipher human speech, he might have recoiled in fear at the ominous mutterings of his master. For you see, dear reader, the man's lips moved in a hushed confession, branding himself a monster for some undisclosed transgression involving a mysterious substance he had unleashed. Such self-condemnation, veiled in cryptic regret, hinted at a dark burden gnawing at the very core of his being. Yet, amidst this somber inner turmoil, Astor, true to his canine nature, remained blissfully ignorant, his snout tracing the familiar contours of a lamppost while he dutifully marked his territory with a well-timed lift of his leg.

Guilt

In the quiet aftermath of World War II, a new chapter unfolded in the Lange household, where a son was welcomed into the world more than a decade after the war's end. They christened him Wolfgang, a nod to the legendary composer Wolfgang Amadeus Mozart, whose musical genius had captivated hearts for centuries.

Gütersloh, a city steeped in history and known for its industrial prowess, provided the backdrop for young Wolfgang's upbringing. Here, amid the hum of machinery and the scent of freshly laundered clothes, his father toiled as a technician while his mother reigned supreme over their modest domain.

Wolfgang, eager to please, eagerly joined his father in tending to the garden and dutifully collecting fallen leaves in the wheelbarrow. Meanwhile, his mother ruled the household with a firm hand, her stern demeanor softened only by the sound of her approving clap when dinner was served.

As Wolfgang grew, so did the family, welcoming a sister during his kindergarten years and a brother later on. Yet, despite the addition of siblings, familial harmony gave way to discord when Wolfgang's academic performance fell short of his father's expectations. Their once-close bond shattered, replaced by simmering resentment and unspoken accusations.

In the eyes of Wolfgang, his father's frequent visits to the local tavern and his mother's domineering presence only fueled his frustration. He longed for the camaraderie they once shared, now lost amidst the weight of unspoken grievances and the burden of unmet expectations.

In the dim light of his tumultuous youth, Wolfgang's path was fraught with adversity and heartache. His father's callous words cast a shadow over his academic pursuits, leading to a premature departure from school after a year of setbacks. Dreams of a promising future in electrical engineering shattered as he was forced to abandon his studies, plagued by subpar performance and unrelenting challenges.

Tragedy struck at the tender age of seventeen when a motorcycle accident left Wolfgang fighting for his life in a hospital bed, his once vibrant spirit dulled by the cruel grip of a double skull fracture. Emerging from the depths of a coma, he battled against persistent concentration issues and relentless headaches, a constant reminder of the fragility of life.

Romance

Amidst the chaos of his tumultuous existence, a flicker of hope emerged in the form of a budding romance. A chance encounter during a dance evening led Wolfgang to the doorstep of love, where awkward coffee dates and hesitant hand-holding marked the tentative beginnings of a meaningful connection. But fate's cruel hand intervened once more as military duty beckoned, tearing him away from his newfound.

The strains of love and duty reached a breaking point when Wolfgang's father, blinded by prejudice, hurled insults at the object of his affection. In a moment of searing rage, Wolfgang confronted his father, his once-forged bond shattered by the weight of resentment and disdain. As his father later lay stricken by a sudden heart attack, Wolfgang's refusal to accompany him to the hospital echoed with the deafening silence of regret. Haunted by the specter of his father's untimely demise, Wolfgang grappled with the burden of guilt, a heavy shroud enveloping his fractured soul.

Upon fulfilling his military duty, Wolfgang found himself drawn to a new path, briefly immersing himself in the world of caring for psychologically troubled men. The experience resonated deeply with him, propelling him through three years of rigorous training as a psychiatric nurse, his academic achievements shining brightly against the backdrop of his tumultuous past. Yet, despite his professional success, Wolfgang remained an enigma, unable to forge meaningful connections beyond the surface in both his academic pursuits and his career.

A beacon of hope emerged in the form of his enduring love for a woman he had known for a decade, offering solace in the midst of his personal struggles. As they embarked on the journey of marriage, they found solace in each other's company, isolated from the world around them. While his wife sought refuge in the pages of books or the glow of the television screen, Wolfgang sought solace in the harmonies of the Concordia men's choir. However, beneath the facade of domestic tranquility, a storm brewed within Wolfgang's soul.

The shadows of suspicion loomed over Wolfgang's professional endeavors, casting a pall over his aspirations. Accusations of theft tainted his reputation, forcing him to part ways with his first job working with vulnerable children. Yet, Wolfgang's plight was not unique, as the dark underbelly of the healthcare industry harbored secrets of deceit and betrayal. The ominous specter of previous incidents like theft, such as those involving Frans H. from the early chapters, cast a chilling shadow over Wolfgang's own troubled path.

In the pages yet to unfold, we delve deeper into Wolfgang's descent into darkness, where the boundaries between right and wrong blur amidst the backdrop of his enigmatic journey.

Descending Into Isolation

Two years into his marriage, Wolfgang embarked on a fresh start at the Westfälische Clinic in Gütersloh, a sprawling institution catering to psychiatry, psychosomatics, and neurology, boasting five hundred beds. Assigned to the General Psychiatry ward, Wolfgang was eager to prove his mettle. However, his enthusiasm grated against the established order as he proposed changes before even settling into his role, earning the ire of his colleagues. Within a mere two years, a new head of department arrived, sparking friction with Wolfgang, resulting in his transfer to the internal ward, a domain predominantly reserved for patients with both mental and physical conditions.

In this realm, Wolfgang found himself in a peculiar position for three reasons: he was the sole male nurse, lacking the supplemental psychosomatic training, and his experience with physically ill patients was limited to his psychiatric education. His assistance was selective, demonstrating favoritism in his attentiveness while showing disdain toward patients grappling with alcohol and drug abuse. Confronted about his behavior, Wolfgang's stoicism was palpable, beads of sweat betraying his discomfort.

Yet, Wolfgang was not alone in his plight. Also his colleagues regarded their domain as the hospital's dumping ground, where the most challenging cases were cast aside. This perception held weight, fueled by an overflow of patients deemed untreatable and the unfortunate practice of adjacent wards unloading their most burdensome cases just before the weekend, met with indifference from the medical staff when nurses voiced their grievances.

Undeterred, Wolfgang labored tirelessly, meticulously managing duty rosters and participating in the staff council. However, his efforts were met with suspicion by his peers, who viewed his desk-bound tasks as a means to shirk his nursing responsibilities. Despite his dedication, Wolfgang's overtures were met with indifference, alienating him further from the staff. Offered a transfer to a specialized psychiatric ward with the promise of a higher salary, Wolfgang declined, steadfast in his commitment to his current post.

As Wolfgang's isolation deepened, a palpable sense of desolation engulfed him, a solitary figure adrift in the abyss of abandonment within the confines of the Westfälische Clinic.

Infertile

In the quiet turmoil of their marriage, the absence of children weighed heavily on Wolfgang's heart and behind closed doors, Wolfgang kept silent about the whispers of theft and the struggles within his workplace, but the couple shared their longing for parenthood, seeking solace in the possibility of a family. Their journey led them to a gynecologist's office, where Wolfgang's world was shattered in early March 1990 with the damning diagnosis: infertile.

The news struck like a hammer, shattering Wolfgang's self-image and dreams of fatherhood. Despite considering adoption and the arrival of their faithful dog, Astor, Wolfgang's despair only deepened. Plunged into a dark abyss of depression, contemplating suicide.

Meanwhile, within the walls of the Westfälische Clinic, a mysterious death unfolded. During the autopsy of a deceased patient, unsettling findings emerged: a suspicious wound on the back of the head and fresh injection marks in the elbow crease. Yet, despite the ominous implications, the body was swiftly released for cremation, leaving behind unanswered questions.

As later the truth unraveled in the courtroom, Wolfgang confessed to a chilling revelation: this was his first murder. The patient, bearing an uncanny resemblance to his father, became the unwitting target of Wolfgang's torment. Injecting a fatal dose of air intravenously, Wolfgang sought to erase his father's memory, but the act only plunged him deeper into darkness.

Haunted by the specter of his crime, Wolfgang confided his sins to the only confidant he trusted, his loyal dog, a silent witness to his descent into the abyss.

Natural Death Certificates

Five weeks passed, marking the onset of a sinister pattern within the sterile walls of the clinic. Two women departed from the realm of the living, their deaths separated by a mere three hours, a macabre sequence unfolding under the watchful gaze of Wolfgang. With a fragmented schedule, Wolfgang embarked on his malevolent mission.

With callous precision, Wolfgang administered a fatal dose of air into the veins of a 92-year-old woman, her transition from life to death a seamless orchestration of his sinister machinations. Unfazed by the gravity of his actions, he notified the family of their loved one's passing before retreating for a long lunchbreak to the sanctity of his own home, consumed by the weight of his transgressions.

Haunted by the specter of his misdeeds, Wolfgang's mind swirled with turmoil, grappling with the consequences of his actions. Yet, amidst the tumult of his thoughts, a chilling resolve emerged, the deadly injections must cease.

Returning to the ward, Wolfgang concealed his malevolent intent behind the facade of caregiving, pushing the coffee trolley along the rows of beds. His gaze fell upon an unsuspecting 82-year-old woman, her fate sealed by the lethal injection he administered. And each time the doctor notes on the form that the death was due to natural causes. As the death toll mounted, Wolfgang's facade of normalcy crumbled, his deeds more and more obscuring behind a veneer of deceit.

Two weeks later, he injects air once again, this time into the vein of a 78-year-old woman. Ten days later, another victim, a 75-year-old man, falls prey to his lethal actions. Barely two months later, an 82-year-old patient becomes his target, followed precisely a month later by a 69-year-old man. Injecting the air first, he then rushes out of the room, only to return five minutes later to find the patient lifeless. And each time, the doctor completes the paperwork, certifying the deaths as natural.

Deadly Fridays

Fridays regularly cast a chilling shadow over Wolfgang's ward, a harbinger of death and suspicion. With alarming regularity, the adjacent wards dispatched their gravely ill patients to Wolfgang's care, a ritual observed with a sense of foreboding by his colleagues. As each Friday unfolded, Wolfgang's presence became synonymous with tragedy, earning him the sardonic nickname 'Angel of Death' amidst whispers of his eerie connection to the demise of patients under his watch.

Especially because the trial of Michaela Roeder, the perpetrator from the previous chapter, is still fresh in everyone's memory. Like the rest, Wolfgang laughs at his nickname.

Five weeks after the dual tragedies that shook the ward, a new crisis emerged, shattering the fragile peace. A patient, struggling for breath, was rushed back to the intensive care unit, triggering a frantic investigation. In a chilling revelation, colleagues stumbled upon discarded vials of a potent muscle relaxant in the trash, absent from any official records. Suspicion loomed heavy over Wolfgang, the only plausible culprit.

As the hospital grappled with mounting unease, six courageous colleagues dared to confront the looming specter of doubt. Their letter to the department head echoed with urgency, a plea to confront the unsettling truths lurking beneath the surface. Their concerns were not unfounded, analysis of the patient's blood revealed damning traces of the muscle relaxant, a sinister clue pointing towards Wolfgang's potential involvement.

Yet, instead of invoking the swift hand of justice, the hospital veiled itself in secrecy, opting for a clandestine internal inquiry. The shadow of suspicion stretched ominously, enveloping Wolfgang in its chilling embrace. Under the scrutiny of his peers, Wolfgang adamantly professed his innocence, a defiant stance amidst the swirling vortex of accusations and doubts.

Ostracized Whistleblowers

Barely a month later, the hospital administration made a startling announcement, the investigation into Wolfgang's alleged misconduct was abruptly terminated. Staff members received the official decree: Wolfgang was no longer under suspicion. However, a peculiar directive followed, an atmosphere of heightened vigilance was to be maintained. This declaration invoked a sense of déjà vu, reminiscent of Martha U.'s ordeal recounted in Chapter 9, where vigilance felt more like waiting for a repeat offender to strike again.

In a baffling twist, Wolfgang graciously thanked the physician for what he deemed a just exoneration. His nonchalant demeanor as he traversed the ward left his colleagues dumbfounded. Yet, beneath the façade of normalcy, a lingering cloud of shame enveloped those who had dared to voice their concerns, akin to the whistleblowers in the preceding chapter. Their tentative accusations had resulted in a colleague being wrongfully implicated, fracturing the unity of the team. While the whistleblowers were ostracized, the rest of the staff rallied openly behind Wolfgang, oblivious to the sinister truth lurking beneath the surface.

Amidst the tumult, a chilling silence descended as the hospital's attention shifted elsewhere. Unnoticed amidst the chaos, the sinister orchestration continued. Three weeks after the harrowing incident that led to a patient's urgent transfer to the intensive care unit, two more souls, aged 87, met their untimely demise. Their deaths, like clockwork, were swiftly attributed to natural causes. Two weeks later, a 97-year-old woman became the latest victim in this macabre charade, her passing cloaked in the same guise of natural death.

Injection Marks

In the case of Wolfgang Lange we see that doctors, unaware of any harm, quite carelessly issue a certificate of natural death. All things considered, they offer healthcare serial killers a recipe for the perfect murder. Beine (1998) discovered in his research that in only one in sixteen crimes the perpetrator was caught because a doctor discovered irregularities. In some cases, doctors even signing a declaration of natural death without seeing the patient, based solely on what the nurse told them.

Amidst the twinkling lights and festive cheer enveloping the Apostelkirche in Gütersloh, the vibrant energy of the Christmas market pulsed through the air on December 14, 1990. Yet, amidst the merry spectacle, a sinister shadow loomed over the psychiatric wards, where Wolfgang Lange's deadly charade unfolded.

Against Wolfgang's protests, an 86-year-old woman, plagued by heart rhythm disturbances, was unceremoniously transferred to his care. Her arrival sparked a fleeting encounter between Wolfgang and the accompanying nurse, whose critical gaze bore down upon him, questioning the absence of a nightstand and his competence in performing an electrocardiogram. With the nurse's departure, Wolfgang seized the opportunity shrouded in the cloak of bustling activity, administering a lethal dose of air to the unsuspecting patient. Not long afterwards he encounters a doctor in the hallway and he says that he did not make an electrocardiogram because the woman is absolutely dead. A sinister scene unfolds as the doctor discovers the patient's lifeless body, lying in repose with hands gently folded, strategically concealing the telltale marks of three injections. Wolfgang, playing the role of the dutiful nurse, meticulously arranges the patient's body before abruptly departing the ward, citing a choral performance awaiting his attendance.

With a professional acumen honed by years of practice, the doctor discerns the faint traces of injections in the delicate crook of the patient's elbow. Memories of a similar occurrence, shrouded in suspicion, resurface, a grim reminder of an unsolved mystery that lingered like a specter in the hospital's annals.

With a sense of urgency, the doctor embarks on a meticulous search, unearthing damning evidence that punctures the veil of Wolfgang's deceit. A discarded syringe, bearing the distinct mark of a butterfly needle for multiple injections, is discovered amidst the medical paraphernalia. In a chilling twist, a tourniquet, a silent accomplice to Wolfgang's lethal machinations, is found concealed within his personal effects.

The pieces of the puzzle fall into place with a sickening clarity, and the doctor wastes no time in summoning the authorities, casting a stark light on the shadowy recesses of Wolfgang's sinister deeds.

But Wolfgang's facade crumbles, and in a chilling revelation during the trial, he confesses to the heinous act, his words echoing with the weight of remorse and unbridled impulse that led to the fatal encounter.

Haunting Confession

In the chill of December, just on the cusp of Christmas and a mere day before his own birthday, Wolfgang finds himself ensnared in the grasp of the law, arrested for a crime he vehemently denies. Yet, as the darkness of night descends, casting shadows over the interrogation room, Wolfgang's resolve begins to falter. Tears betraying his stoic facade, he succumbs to the weight of guilt and confesses to the woman's murder.

His admission shocks the investigators, who pry into his motivations. With a trembling voice, Wolfgang reveals a chilling plot: he sought to exacerbate the woman's condition, orchestrating her transfer to the intensive care unit to alleviate his own burdensome workload. It's a confession that chills the marrow, revealing the depths of his callousness.

But Wolfgang's tale doesn't end there. In the aftermath of his initial confession, a flicker of remorse prompts him to amend his statement, seeking solace in the counsel of his mother and legal advisor. It's during this poignant moment of introspection that Wolfgang unveils a harrowing truth: he's responsible for the deaths of not one, not two, but approximately fourteen patients.

A Jolt of Recognition

Meanwhile, amidst the turmoil, psychiatrist and psychotherapist Karl Heinz Beine, upon reading about Wolfgang's arrest, experiences a jolt of recognition. Memories of their shared past in the halls of the hospital flood his mind, mingling with a sense of disbelief at Wolfgang's descent into darkness. Yet, amidst the shock, a determination takes root within Beine, a resolve to unearth the unsettling truth lurking within the shadows of the healthcare system. He decided to do research, resulting in the book eight years later: *Sehen, Hören, Schweigen, Patientstötungen und active Sterbehilfe*, (1998). He discovers that Wolfgang is far from the only staff member in a healthcare facility who kills patients and that there is a dire need to publicize this subject.

As the investigation deepens in Gütersloh, uncovering a staggering tally of suspicious deaths, Wolfgang's reign of terror is brought to light. Charged with ten murders, a grim testament to the depths of his depravity, Wolfgang's story serves as a chilling reminder of the darkness that can lurk behind the sterile facade of a hospital ward.

Bow Tie

As the courtroom doors swing open, revealing the figure of the defendant, all eyes turn towards Wolfgang, his presence a stark contrast to the solemn surroundings. Clad in a crisp suit adorned with a bow tie, his appearance belies the gravity of the charges laid against him. With a boyish countenance marred by a smattering of chin hairs, reminiscent of a boy in a man's body.

In a hushed courtroom, Wolfgang's voice breaks the silence, his words tinged with a haunting confession that reverberates through the chamber. 'I never entered a patient's room with premeditation,' he admits, his tone fraught with a remorseful cadence. 'At times, I didn't even know their names. But when faced with a patient trapped in a hopeless plight, I found myself unable to resist the urge to act.' Words which heavily hang in the air.

The presiding judge, with a keen gaze honed by years of adjudicating the complexities of human nature, poses a poignant question that cuts to the heart of the matter. 'Why, then, did you habitually carry a sterile 20-cc syringe and a butterfly needle?'

Wolfgang shrugs.

A fellow healthcare worker takes the stand, casting a damning light on Wolfgang's actions. Recounting an unsettling incident from 1989, they describe Wolfgang's ominous prediction of three patients' impending demise during a shift change. The chilling nonchalance with which Wolfgang declared 'Mission accomplished' the following morning. He had also noticed that Wolfgang was always the first to offer help after death when laying down a patient and how rudely Wolfgang handled the corpse. For example, the suspect once said shortly after a death: 'There, we don't have to wash this anymore, he can go straight into his coffin'. Leaving an indelible impression, a stark reminder of the sinister undercurrents lurking beneath the facade of compassion.

The Shattered Self

In the annals of criminal psychology, the case of Wolfgang Lange stands as a chilling testament to the intricate complexities of the human mind. As the courtroom becomes a stage for his psychological unraveling, experts dissect the enigma of his psyche, revealing a narrative fraught with despair and desperation.

Described as possessing above-average intellect but marred by only moderate social development, Wolfgang's inner turmoil is laid bare. At the crux of his affliction lies a pre-suicidal syndrome, a haunting specter that shadows his every move. It's a syndrome born from a relentless barrage of life's adversities, compounded by the devastating revelation of his infertility, a cruel blow that shattered his fragile sense of self.

Within this maelstrom of despair, the concept of projective identification emerges as a pivotal mechanism. Wolfgang, grappling with his own death wish, unwittingly projected this existential anguish onto his unsuspecting patients, a twisted manifestation of his inner torment.

Yet, the labyrinthine depths of Wolfgang's psyche reveal more than mere projection. Three distinct factors intertwine to shape his descent into darkness: one, a profound sense of inadequacy, two, festering rage, and three, an inexorable compulsion. Struggling beneath the weight of his own perceived worthlessness, Wolfgang perceived every slight, real or imagined, as a personal affront, a wound that festered, fueling a tempest of rage.

In a desperate bid to reclaim a semblance of control, Wolfgang sought solace in violence, a twisted attempt to bolster his crumbling self-worth. Each life extinguished served as a fleeting reprieve, a momentary respite from the relentless onslaught of his inner demons.

It cannot be ruled out that he tried to boost his low self-esteem with his act, feeling more imposing by carrying a secret. Every time he killed someone, a piece of his sense of self died, lowering the threshold for striking again.

However, in the eyes of experts following strict guidelines, Wolfgang Lange is deemed fully responsible for his actions during his spree of murders.

The defense attorneys representing Wolfgang Lange find themselves facing a daunting task in their plea. They emphasize their client's isolated nature within the department and the longstanding unresolved conflicts that plagued the environment. Additionally, drawing parallels to the trial of Michaela Roeder detailed in the previous chapter, they acknowledge their client's inability to craft a motive rooted in compassion.

In a decisive ruling, the judge delivers a sentence of ten counts of manslaughter, condemning Wolfgang Lange to a fifteen-year term behind bars. While some may perceive this as lenient, especially given the absence of mitigating factors, the judge adamantly rejects the notion that the convicted is a sadistic killer. Furthermore, the medical director of the Westfälische Klinik faces scrutiny for neglecting to involve law enforcement when suspicions arose in March 1990, following the discovery of unexplained head injuries and injection marks on a patient, coupled with the subsequent finding of four empty ampoules, which raised serious concerns regarding Wolfgang.

Wolfgang Lange has since been released and now resides under an assumed identity.

15.

A disillusioned youth

Rudi Paul Zimmermann, Germany, 1970

Daring

In the chill of November 1970, two aspiring caregivers stepped into the hallowed halls of the German Evangelical Altenheim in Wupperfeld. Little did they know, their journey into the world of elder care would be fraught with darkness and deceit.

Their hearts heavy with the burden of truth they approached their instructor reporting the misconduct of the nursing manager, hoping for solace and guidance. Instead, they were met with a chilling rebuke, a warning to silence their tongues if they wished to pass their exams unscathed. 'Leave the rest to God', they were told, as if divine intervention could rectify the sins they had uncovered.

But one among them refused to heed such hollow counsel. With courage in her heart and determination in her eyes, she sought out the sanctuary of the director's office. There, she laid bare the atrocities committed by Herr Rudi, the nursing manager whose shadow loomed over the facility like a specter of despair.

She spoke of the orders to administer potent sedatives to helpless residents, of medications administered in secrecy, defying all medical protocol. She recounted tales of cruelty and callousness, of rough hands and rougher words that left scars deeper than any physical wound.

And when the director's ears were filled with the echoes of her words, he knew that action must be taken. With a heavy heart but a steely resolve, he cast Herr Rudi out into the cold, his reign of terror brought to a swift and decisive end.

But justice, as always, is a fickle mistress. Herr Rudi remained steadfast in his denial, a wolf in sheep's clothing clinging to the last vestiges of his innocence.

Yet amidst the darkness, a glimmer of hope shines through. For in the bravery of those two caregivers lies a testament to the resilience of the human spirit, a reminder that even in the face of unspeakable evil, there are those who will stand up and speak out, fighting for justice in a world gone awry.

Favorite Rabbit

In the humble beginnings of 1929, Rudi was born amidst the backdrop of a modest working-class household, nestled as the second of four siblings. His early years were unremarkable, drifting through school with average marks and blending seamlessly with his peers.

Behind the facade of familial harmony lay a discordant note, his father's domineering presence. While his mother, the quintessential homemaker, toiled tirelessly to maintain a facade of familial unity, Rudi's relationship with her remained a mystery. Meanwhile, his father, a municipal worker staunchly opposed to the rising tide of National Socialism, clashed ideologically with his devoutly religious wife.

Yet, it was a single, brutal act that shattered the fragile peace within their home, the callous slaughter of Rudi's cherished pet rabbit, a cruel blow that severed the bond between father and son irreparably.

As the clouds of war loomed over Germany, Rudi's adolescent years were marked by a disturbing fascination with violence. Alongside his comrades, he reveled in the hunt for downed Allied pilots, indulging in acts of brutality that foreshadowed the darkness lurking within.

At the tender age of fifteen, Rudi was seduced by the siren song of National Socialism, casting aside his education to join the ranks of the Hitler Youth. His pocket money, painstakingly saved, he bought the book *Mein Kampf,* a tome that would shape his burgeoning ideology.

In the shadow of impending conflict, Rudi's descent into darkness had begun, setting the stage for a chilling narrative of manipulation, violence, and the inexorable march towards a fate intertwined with the darkest chapters of history.

In the annals of wartime history, Rudi's tale unfolds like a dark odyssey through the depths of human suffering and survival. Enlisting in the Waffen-SS, Rudi is thrust into the heart of chaos, tasked with clandestine operations behind enemy lines. His orders are clear: sabotage at any cost, even if it means the swift execution of foes and comrades alike. Amidst the carnage, Rudi emerges battered but alive, a testament to his resilience in the face of relentless adversity. Yet, his respite is short-lived as he is inevitably captured, becoming a prisoner of war.

Through a stroke of luck and the cunning of a few influential officers, Rudi secures his release with forged documents in hand. His journey home is a tortuous one, fraught with the ghosts of his past and the grim reality of a world forever changed by war. Returning to a fractured family, Rudi is met with the bitter truth: his mother, kin, and friends have all perished in the turmoil of conflict.

Haunted by his wartime experiences, Rudi's emotions lie buried beneath layers of trauma, emerging only in the most extreme circumstances. It is amidst this emotional numbness that he finds solace in the field of healthcare, drawn to the altruistic desire to aid others, a guidepost amid the darkness that shrouds his soul. As he embarks on the arduous path of nursing training, Rudi dares to believe that perhaps, amidst the wreckage of his past, there lies a glimmer of redemption and purpose.

Tempestuous

In the tumultuous tapestry of Rudi's life, both his professional journey and personal relationships paint a picture of turbulence and change, with 23 years bearing witness to 25 different positions and three marriages, yielding eight children along the way.

Firstly, his career. At the tender age of 21, Rudi's path intersects with a Christian youth circle, igniting a fervor within him. Driven by a desire to serve, he sets his sights on becoming a deacon, embarking on the rigorous training required, all while pursuing his studies in nursing.

But Rudi's journey towards spiritual fulfillment proves to be a labyrinth fraught with disappointment. Despite his fervent efforts, a cloud of disapproval descends upon him, shrouding his aspirations in darkness. His superiors deliver a damning verdict, severing his path to ordination as a deacon and compelling him to depart. Undeterred by rejection, Rudi defiantly clings to his aspirations, yet he purchases a toga and continues to call himself a deacon.

As a parish assistant in various churches and a transient presence in numerous healthcare facilities, Rudi's tenure is marked by instability and discord. His employment is a series of short-lived engagements, punctuated by conflicts and breaches of authority that force him to move on time and again. However, his professional missteps pale in comparison to the dark shadow of his criminal record, which includes convictions for theft, fraud, and even disturbing reports of mistreatment of vulnerable children.

But it is in the realm of personal relationships where Rudi's tumultuous nature truly shines. His romantic entanglements are fraught with drama and heartbreak, characterized by a pattern of abandonment and abuse. His first marriage, to a fellow nurse, ends in disappointment, leading him to seek solace in the arms of a younger woman. Their union, marked by manipulation and violence, unravels, only for Rudi to embark on yet another ill-fated affair, culminating in another marriage.

Despite the chaos that swirls around him, Rudi's legacy as a father is marred by neglect and abandonment. His children, scattered across multiple relationships, are left to navigate the complexities of life without the guidance and support of a loving parent. And as Rudi's tangled web of deceit and betrayal unravels, it becomes clear that his journey is a cautionary tale of the consequences of unchecked ambition and the destructive power of unchecked desire.

Megalomaniacal

In the heart of the Evangelical Altenheim, a storm is brewing. A judicial inquiry unfolds, unraveling a web of manipulation and deceit woven by none other than Rudi himself.

As investigators piece together the puzzle, a chilling narrative emerges from the whispers of former staff members. Rudi's brief stint at the institution, spanning from August 1970 to January 1971, leaves a trail of destruction in its wake.

With a megalomaniacal fervor, Rudi remakes the landscape of the institution to suit his whims. Office renovations are just the beginning; he proceeds to order the destruction of kitchen supplies under the guise of spoilage. Residents are forcibly relocated, their belongings carelessly tossed out of windows like discarded memories.

Under the guise of authority, Rudi enforces a code of silence among staff, dictating their every move. In a brazen display of power, he mandates that residents can only seek medical attention from physicians of his choosing, disregarding their longstanding relationships with their own GP's.

But Rudi's ambitions know no bounds. With a cunning hand, he orchestrates the creation of a secret haven within the facility, stocked with a clandestine supply of medications procured through dubious means. The appointed physician, swayed by Rudi's charisma, unwittingly becomes a pawn in his game, enabling his unchecked access to opiates.

In this dark enclave, Rudi's delusions of grandeur reach new heights. Equipped with medical tools fit for a surgical theater, he wields his authority with a callous disregard for the lives in his care. Behind closed doors, the facade of compassion crumbles, revealing a man consumed by his own thirst for control.

As the investigation unfolds, the truth behind Rudi's reign of terror begins to surface, painting a portrait of a man driven by a dangerous cocktail of power and delusion. And in the shadows of the Evangelical Altenheim, the echoes of his misdeeds reverberate, leaving a trail of devastation in their wake.

Objects

As Rudi stepped into his new role, the atmosphere at the institution began to shift. Initially, there were two nurses working alongside the caregivers, but Rudi's arrival heralded a change that rattled the foundation of the facility.

The first nurse, unimpressed by Rudi's so-called improvements, dares to voice her concerns. In response, Rudi unleashes a tirade reminiscent of a petulant child denied their way. He threatens the nurse with swift retribution, forcing her to visit the company doctor under threat of termination. The nurse complies, only to find herself sidelined on sick leave until the end of 1970, and ultimately dismissed.

With the departure of the second nurse, Rudi's unchecked behavior spirals further out of control. His words become weapons, laced with cruelty and disregard for the dignity of the residents. He shows callous indifference to the deceased, treating them as little more than objects to be discarded at will.

But Rudi's transgressions extend beyond mere words. His actions paint a chilling portrait of a man unhinged. He disappears without explanation, leaving a wake of confusion and fear in his path. His interactions with vulnerable residents cross the line into outright abuse, leaving them traumatized and vulnerable.

Amidst the chaos, whispers of suspicion begin to circulate. At least six deaths occur under questionable circumstances, casting a shadow of doubt over Rudi's actions.

As the investigation unfolds, the detectives are forced to confront the chilling truth: they are dealing with a man whose delusions of grandeur are matched only by his capacity for cruelty. In the face of such darkness, they must navigate a treacherous path, unraveling the twisted web of Rudi's madness before more lives are lost.

Coincidence

Five months after departing the Evangelical Altenheim, Rudi resurfaces in the workforce, this time as a nursing coordinator at the Sint Elisabeth Hospital in Neviges. As fate would have it, amidst the ongoing judicial inquiry into his previous actions, references are conveniently overlooked.

Yet, it doesn't take long for the whispers of discontent to resurface. At a departmental meeting, Rudi faces criticism for his questionable handling of patient records. The ensuing scrutiny prompts a swift reassignment to the ambulance service, a precautionary measure taken by the responsible doctor, who seems eager to sweep any potential issues under the rug.

Unwilling to face further scrutiny, Rudi opts to tender his resignation in March of that year.

Subsequent investigations paint a disturbing picture of Rudi's tenure at the Sint Elisabeth Hospital. Allegations surface suggesting Rudi's involvement in questionable medical practices, including administering injections to patients without proper authorization.

What surprises the detectives most is the complimentary testimonial that Rudi received upon his departure, praising his exceptional helpfulness, great organizational skills, collegiality and professional knowledge.

Two years later, the preliminary judicial investigation into the report in the first institution has still not been completed. The original statements of the energetic care worker have not been confirmed by anyone. And nothing prevents Rudi from accepting a next position in a third institution. This time he is appointed as head nurse in the men's wing at the Hattingen-Blankenstein hospital.

Within five months, disaster struck once again. Fate intervened in the form of the fiancée of the aspiring caregiver who first sounded the alarm at the initial institution, the Evangelical Altenheim in Wupperfeld. Little did anyone know, her fiancée was now employed at the very hospital where the sinister saga would unfold.

Rumors swirled as whispers of a box of opiates found in Rudi's possession reached the ears of the fiancée. With a sinking feeling, he realized the gravity of the situation. And Rudi's employment was swiftly terminated.

As authorities combed through his office, they unearthed a trove of 170 ampoules of opiates and textbooks from doctors who had once praised Rudi. Stoically, Rudi denied any wrongdoing, his façade of composure barely concealing the depths of his deception. The judicial investigation lasted two and a half years more and after having been employed by two more hospitals, Rudi Z. was eventually arrested.

When his precise actions are later examined, his start in the third setting is also striking.

His charismatic charm belied a chilling reality as he seamlessly ingratiated himself with colleagues and patients alike. With a silver tongue, he convinced patients of his medical expertise, only to betray their trust with a needle and a dose of deadly medication.

A search of his home revealed a cache of narcotics and medical supplies fit for an emergency ward. As the investigation deepened, the tally of victims rose, culminating in a staggering indictment: nine lives lost, a testament to Rudi's reign of terror across three institutions.

Biting Chill

It was a full six years after the apprentice caregiver sounded the alarm that the trial began in the spring of 1976 at the district court of Wuppertal, stretching through the heat of summer and delving into the sinister web woven by Rudi.

The proceedings opened with the six charges stemming from his tenure at the Evangelical nursing home in Wupperfeld. It was during those short three and a half months that Rudi's dark intentions first surfaced. A resident whispered to a visitor of Herr Rudi's frequent injections. Two days later, the resident was inexplicably gone.

As Rudi sat stoically in the defendant's chair, his memory of the events conveniently faded. But the judge saw through the facade, recognizing Rudi's calculated attempts to hasten the demise of his troublesome patient.

Days turned into weeks, and another tragedy unfolded. A vigilant staff member witnessed Rudi administering intravenous fluid to a patient, preemptively covering the body before the last breath had even left her lips. While the specifics of the lethal concoction remained elusive, the act of administering unauthorized injections cast a damning shadow over Rudi's actions.

The pattern repeated with a chilling predictability as a third victim succumbed under similar circumstances. Rudi's cavalier attitude, coupled with his disturbingly accurate predictions of death, painted a picture of a man unburdened by remorse.

Though the exact cause of death remained shrouded in ambiguity, the undeniable truth emerged: Rudi had inflicted intentional harm.

Later still, another haunting episode unfolded in the chilling saga. One of the residents lay unresponsive, unable to be awakened. When confronted by a nurse, Rudi delivered a callous pronouncement: the woman no longer needed sustenance, for she would soon be resting in the embrace of heaven, receiving only medication henceforth. With a cruel disregard for the season, he flung open the windows wide, exposing the frail figure to the biting chill of November. The following morning, two volunteers were met with a ghastly sight: the elderly woman still clung to life, her extremities cold and blue. Without hesitation, Rudi administered a potent sedative intravenously, proclaiming that the resident's time had come. His grim prophecy proved eerily accurate as the woman succumbed to the lethal injection, leaving the volunteers stunned witnesses to the unfolding tragedy. While the specter of death by hypothermia loomed, the court grappled with the lack of concrete evidence and the elusive nature of determining the extent of the administered overdose.

Drowning

In early 1971, the fifth inexplicable death sent shockwaves. Following an injection from Rudi, a woman faltered, her condition deteriorating rapidly. Before she could regain her bearings, Rudi brandished yet another syringe, poised to deliver another deadly dose. True to form, the doctor denied any involvement in prescribing medication. That evening, a chilling phone call from Rudi to the woman's daughter forewarned of her mother's imminent demise. In a macabre display of his twisted methods, Rudi sought to demonstrate the severity of the situation to the grieving family. With a callous disregard for human life, he casually manipulated the woman's arm, only to drop it with a thud. As the woman breathed her last breath, Rudi callously suggested to the attending doctor a diagnosis of stroke, a fabrication that was readily accepted and documented. The court left no room for doubt: this victim had met her untimely end at the hands of Rudi's deadly injections.

The chilling series of events continued to unfold with the final attempt at murder in the initial institution occurring just four days later. A resident, fearing for her life, confided in her niece about Rudi's sinister intentions, claiming he was administering 'death pills' because she was next in line to die. It was a vigilant caregiver who stumbled upon the woman unconscious in her bed, an empty ampoule of antipsychotic medication lying nearby. With a cold and calculated demeanor, Rudi entered the room and proceeded to inject the woman with not one, but two different types of sleeping pills. Miraculously, later that same afternoon, the decisive actions of a staff member led to the woman's recovery. A doctor confirmed that the dosage of medication administered could have been lethal.

Meanwhile, on the very day Rudi commenced his employment at the second institution in June 1971, suspicions arose surrounding the death of a woman admitted with a complicated leg fracture. Just four weeks later, visitors were horrified to find her in a dazed state. Rudi's explanation was as chilling as it was callous: the woman had supposedly become addicted to opiates and required escalating doses. That evening, tragedy struck as the patient drowned in her bath. Rudi, ever the manipulator, warned a colleague to keep quiet, despite the apparent accident. However, the court saw through the facade, determining that the woman's death was a result of drowning induced by an injection that left her in a semi-comatose state.

In the final institution where Rudi wielded his deadly influence, two more suspicious deaths occurred. Despite the mounting evidence, both charges were ultimately dropped due to a lack of concrete proof. Once again, doctors chalked up the deaths to natural causes, leaving a lingering sense of injustice in their wake.

Fully Accountable

Between the ages of 39 and 41, Rudi embarks on a dark journey of crime. Physically fit, with average intelligence and a silver tongue, he is also culturally refined. But where does it all go so drastically awry?

According to psychiatric and psychological evaluations, Rudi is diagnosed with a neurotic, psychopathic personality. Yet, this diagnosis does not absolve him of responsibility for his actions. His already fragile sense of identity crumbles further when his aspirations of becoming a deacon are dashed. The longed-for approval from his father for his nursing credentials remains elusive, shattered by his father's untimely death a year prior. Unable to reconcile his childish fantasies of grandeur with reality, Rudi begins to assert himself with increasing recklessness.

In the midst of his delusions of grandeur, Rudi loses touch with professional ethics, soaring above the boundaries of acceptable behavior. His actions become dictated by his own idealized self-image, with little regard for the opinions of others. In his own opinion, he is the epitome of reliability, composure, and control, seamlessly fitting into any social group. And even believes himself to be the ideal husband and father.

From the conclusion of this case, no one was taken aback. The judge deemed Rudi fully responsible and sentenced him to life in prison for three counts of murder, three attempted murders, and premeditated grievous bodily harm. According to the court, Rudi prioritized his ambition and compulsive need for order over the lives of challenging patients. Such sinister and unacceptable behavior warranted the severest punishment, especially given Rudi's knowledge as a nurse of the lethal effects of the medications he administered.

Similar to the tales of Irene Becker, Kristen Gilbert, and Beverley Allitt in earlier chapters, Rudi's method of patient murder involved considerable risk. He administered unauthorized medications and mistreated patients right under everyone's noses, increasing the chances of discovery. This daring is a shared trait among serial killers, as if they seek an extra thrill as the risk of getting caught grows. In contrast, Stephan Letter, the perpetrator in the following chapter who took the lives of numerous patients, had the courtesy to politely ask visiting family members to step out into the hallway before committing his crimes.

16.

On deaf ears

Stephan Letter, Germany, 2003

A Soldier's Nightmare

In the quiet halls of the Kliniken Oberallgäu, a young Bundeswehr soldier battles not only her physical wounds but also the haunting shadows of doubt that threaten to engulf her sanity.

At just 22 years old, she lies confined to the sterile confines of the hospital's internal department, a casualty of a fall that left her battered and broken. Yet, as she bravely fights to reclaim her strength, a sinister presence lurks in the shadows, waiting to strike.

It begins innocently enough, with the gentle hum of medical equipment and the soft footsteps of caring nurses. But when a towering figure, shrouded in mystery, materializes at her bedside, the soldier's world is plunged into darkness. With a swift and calculated hand, the enigmatic stranger administers a lethal dose of liquid into her IV tube, sending her spiraling into unconsciousness.

As she awakens, disoriented and bewildered, the soldier's mind races with fear and uncertainty. Desperate for answers, she confides in the attending physician, recounting the chilling encounter with a trembling voice. Yet, her pleas for validation fall on deaf ears as skepticism clouds the doctor's judgment.

But the woman begs him to please have her blood examined in the laboratory just to be sure. The doctor wants nothing to do with this, but promises to ask the male nurse for an explanation. However, since Stephan vehemently denies ever having been in her room, the doctor tells the patient that she must have imagined the whole thing, and that's the end of it. But did the soldier really imagine the incident?

Tragic Tale

From the very beginning, Stephan Letter's life is shrouded in darkness, his innocence tainted by the twisted whims of fate that grip him even before he draws his first breath.

Born into a world of turmoil, his mother's paranoid convictions cast a sinister shadow over his prenatal existence. Convinced that her unborn child is flawed, she subjects herself to an astonishing thirteen ultrasounds, a desperate attempt to validate her unfounded fears. It's a chilling echo of the infamous Munchausen by Proxy syndrome, a harbinger of the chaos that awaits young Stephan.

As he enters the world, his arrival heralds not joy but a continuation of his mother's obsessive quest for attention. From the quaint town of Herdecke in Northwest Germany, she embarks on a relentless journey, traversing vast distances in pursuit of doctors who will affirm her darkest suspicions. For Stephan, this means enduring a barrage of invasive tests and painful examinations, all orchestrated by a mother consumed by her own delusions.

But the true tragedy unfolds with the dissolution of his parents' marriage when Stephan is just three and a half years old. Cast adrift in a sea of dysfunction, he becomes a pawn in a bitter custody battle, torn between a father desperate to protect him and a mother consumed by her own twisted obsessions.

At the tender age of four, his behavior at kindergarten paints him as a small despot, leading to his referral to a child psychologist for treatment of behavioral issues. It's a stark revelation of the emotional neglect that has clouded his young life.

His mother, steadfast in her conviction that Stephan is intellectually disabled, enrolls him in a school for mentally handicapped children, perpetuating the cycle of misunderstanding and isolation that grips the young boy's world.

When his father emerges victorious in the custody battle, a scene of heartbreak unfolds. Accompanied by a bailiff, he arrives to claim his son, only to be met with resistance from the frightened seven-year-old who guards the sanctuary of his home. In a moment fraught with anguish, Stephan's father reluctantly retreats, leaving the child torn between loyalty to both parents.

Substitute

Reflecting on this pivotal moment in later years, Stephan laments, 'I was, in any case, the loser. Whichever step I took, I would certainly lose one of my two parents.'

In the tumultuous chapters of Stephan Letter's life, each turn of fate leaves behind shattered promises and unfulfilled dreams, painting a portrait of a young man caught in the tangled web of circumstance and choice.

Now under the roof of his father, Stephan walks the path of a typical student, yet his refuge lies not in books or friends, but in the solace of food. Pouring his entire allowance into sugary treats, he finds comfort in indulgence, his frame expanding as a result. When taunts of 'fat guy' echo through the school halls, Stephan's response is swift and violent, a glimpse into the simmering turmoil within.

Despite his struggles, Stephan navigates the corridors of high school with relative ease. But as he stands on the brink of adulthood at sixteen, a new opportunity beckons, a chance to serve with the Youth Red Cross's rescue brigade. It's here that Stephan discovers a sense of purpose, a calling to aid those in need that ignites a flicker of hope amidst the darkness.

Yet, just as his path seems set, the call to military service disrupts his fragile equilibrium. Although it may seem strange in light of his later actions, killing is not something he can stomach, so he opts for alternative civilian service, transporting the elderly in the quaint streets of Ludwigsburg. It's a noble task that brings him solace, but also forces him to confront the harsh realities of aging and mortality.

Amidst the chaos of duty and devotion, Stephan makes a solemn vow to his father, a promise to shield him from the cold confines of a nursing home. But as the sands of time slip through his fingers, Stephan grapples with the bitter truth that some promises are destined to remain unfulfilled, leaving behind only the echoes of shattered dreams and the weight of regret.

Girlfriend

As Stephan completes his alternative civilian service, he embarks on a journey into the world of nursing, enrolling in a program at a local hospital where he now resides in the dormitories. Yet, behind the facade of normalcy lies a tumultuous existence, where Stephan's quick temper and clashes with authority figures hint at deeper psychological struggles.

Weekends bring no respite for Stephan, as he wanders the empty halls of the dormitory, adrift in a sea of uncertainty. It is here that he encounters his girlfriend, a troubled soul with a harrowing past. She speaks of unspeakable traumas inflicted by her own family members and trusted physicians, tales that hint at a fragile psyche teetering.

Despite her hesitance to engage in physical intimacy, Stephan finds himself inexplicably drawn to her, tethered to her by an invisible thread of shared pain and unspoken secrets.

Stephan's father, a silent observer to the unfolding drama, sees echoes of his ex-wife in his son's girlfriend: the same desperate plea for attention, the same melancholic tone that echoes through the corridors of their troubled past.

As Stephan dreams of a future filled with the familiar aspirations of marriage, children, and a home nestled in the picturesque Allgäu Alps, his girlfriend's desires intertwine with his own, leading them down a path fraught with uncertainty and hidden dangers.

In the quiet halls of Klinikum Kempten in Oberallgäu, a sinister presence lurks, hidden behind the façade of medical care. Stephan Letter, a man with a troubled past and a chilling disposition, weaves a web of deception and death in the heart of the hospital.

As his girlfriend is employed in the pediatric department, Stephan secures a position in the urological wing. Yet, his arrival is not met with open arms but rather a watchful eye. His colleagues soon take note of his antisocial behavior and unprofessional conduct towards patients, leading to his swift dismissal after a mere four months.

Undeterred, Stephan, now 25, finds himself in the internal medicine department of a hospital in Sonthofen, a stone's throw away from the couple's residence. It is in this hospital that the Bundeswehr soldier will be admitted four months later.

Little do his colleagues know that a deadly storm is brewing, one that will shatter the lives of those who cross his path.

Within weeks of his employment, Stephan commits his first murder, a chilling act of violence against an 82-year-old man admitted for a brain hemorrhage. But this is just the beginning of a reign of terror that will grip the hospital in fear.

Months later, a distressed 84-year-old cancer patient reaches out to her son, terrified by the presence of a malevolent figure she calls 'a male nurse who lurks in the shadows', threatening her very existence. Despite her pleas for help, her cries go unanswered, and the next day, she is found lifeless, her death attributed to internal complications by unsuspecting doctors.

Haunting Nightshift

In the quiet solitude of a Sonthofen home, a phone call shatters the evening stillness on June 23, 2004. It's a call no one expects, least of all the woman preparing to draw her curtains against the encroaching darkness. It's her sister on the line, bearing news of their mother's worsening condition.

Together, they rush to the hospital, arriving in the dimly lit hallway of the internal medicine department just past ten o'clock. The air is heavy with anticipation as they step into the hushed corridor, their footsteps echoing in the silence.

But as they approach their mother's room, a stout figure emerges, a familiar face known for his compassion and care. Yet tonight, his demeanor is tense, his voice a hushed command as he urges them to silence for fear of disturbing their mother's roommate.

Bewildered, the sisters watch him disappear into the darkness, leaving them standing in the hallway, their questions unanswered and their hearts heavy with unease.

As they finally enter their mother's room, their relief turns to dread as they find her lying limp and frail, her voice a mere whisper amidst the stillness of the night.

In the darkness of that fateful night in Sonthofen, the sisters are left to grapple with the haunting mystery of what truly transpired behind closed doors.

In the hushed stillness of a hospital room, the mother lies silent, her daughters by her side, their hearts heavy with dread. They exchange a solemn pact, one of them will stay, a silent sentinel, while the other departs to fetch the necessities of home.

The choice falls upon the sister who can drive, her hands trembling as she navigates the familiar streets under the cloak of night. And then, a sudden interruption, the shrill ring of her mobile phone, piercing the darkness like an omen of impending tragedy.

On the other end of the line, a voice she knows all too well, the nurse from the hospital, his words chilling in their brevity. 'The doctor has requested me to inform you that your mother has suffered a heart attack.'

Racing back to the hospital, she arrives to find the room cloaked in shadows, the nurse's comforting arm around her shoulders, his words a cold comfort in the face of loss.

Paella

But tragedy strikes again, barely a fortnight later, as a vibrant soul, full of life and laughter, is silenced forever. A 73-year-old immigrant from Spain, her dreams of a family feast shattered by the cold grip of death. During the evening visiting hours, she chats animatedly with her nephews. Making plans to make a large pan of paella before going on vacation to Spain, insisting that everyone must come and eat. Making it never back to her homeland, as she is found lifeless in bed shortly after sunrise.

Stephan Letter ultimately murders an estimated thirty patients at irregular intervals.

In late July 2004, a staff member discovers a large quantity of medication missing. It's not until a month later that the police are notified and an investigation begins. This delay gives Stephan the opportunity to assist three of his final victims on three consecutive days.

Trembling Hands

In the tranquil embrace of their quaint village, Stephan and his girlfriend seamlessly meld into the tapestry of rural life. Their charming cottage, nestled amidst towering pines and distant peaks, belies the sinister shadows lurking beneath their facade.

To the unsuspecting eye, they are the epitome of normalcy: neatly stacked firewood in the garden, friendly nods exchanged with neighbors.

Stephan, with his unassuming demeanor, conceals a chilling secret, his involvement in illicit activities within the hospital where he works. Meanwhile, his girlfriend's erratic behavior raises eyebrows among the villagers. Her screams and fainting spells, a haunting echo of past traumas, remain shrouded in mystery. In order to be able to do something, Stephan administers sedatives to his girlfriend, which he stole from the Klinikum.

As the investigative team of detectives assembles, the truth begins to unravel. Through meticulous analysis of medication records and duty schedules, leading them straight to nurse Stephan. A search of his home reveals a cache of stolen medications, a shocking revelation of his sinister intentions.

Though the detectives refrain from explicitly implicating him in the murders, the evidence speaks volumes. Stephan's calm facade crumbles as he is escorted to the police station, his carefully constructed world collapsing around him.

As he steps into the interrogation room, Stephan Letter's demeanor betrays the weight of his hidden secrets. With a heavy heart and trembling hands, he makes a shocking revelation to the detectives, admitting to the cold-blooded murder of ten gravely ill patients, their lives extinguished by a deadly concoction of medications. The detectives, hardened by years of experience, are momentarily stunned by his chilling confession, a confession that reverberates with the echoes of his sinister deeds.

Intriguingly, Stephan vividly recalls the details of his first murder, a moment etched in his memory with unnerving clarity. It's a revelation that captivates the attention of the prosecutor, who later highlights its significance in the courtroom.

Mirror Image

To unravel the complexities of Stephan's psyche, we delve into the insights of renowned researcher Karl Heinz Beine. According to him, the first murder of a serial killer is akin to the intoxicating rush of a 'normal' person's first experience of falling in love. It's an act that offers the greatest satisfaction, fueling an insatiable desire to replicate and exceed the initial thrill with each subsequent kill. Yet, this insatiable urge does not strip the killer of their ability to make calculated decisions. Instead, pauses in their killing spree may occur when the fear of discovery looms large or when the killer is momentarily 'distracted' by external factors.

During the second interrogation, Stephan expresses a sense of relief at finally unburdening himself. He meticulously details his crimes in a six-page confession, delving into the twisted dynamics of his relationship with his girlfriend. In his eyes, she becomes a mirror of his disturbed mother,

her volatile outbursts and tyrannical behavior serving as catalysts for his descent into darkness. As the layers of deception are peeled away, Stephan Letter's confession unveils the chilling depths of his depravity, leaving a haunting imprint on all who encounter his twisted tale.

'How could he have operated under our very noses, extinguishing lives with such impunity?' The question hangs heavily in the minds of those who knew him, as they grapple with the unsettling revelation that Stephan's sinister deeds went unnoticed amidst the bustling corridors.

Amidst the bewildering aftermath, a troubling pattern emerges, a pattern of ignored complaints and overlooked warning signs. Colleagues had voiced concerns about nurse Stephan's behavior, yet their pleas fell on deaf ears, shielded by the protective veil of the nursing department. And indeed, it is striking that in this case it is not the epidemic of deaths that stands out, but the missing medicines.

Stephan's demeanor, characterized by alternating moments of callousness and compassion, paints a perplexing portrait of a man with two faces. Behind his affable facade lurked a dark undercurrent of disregard for professional boundaries, evidenced by his inappropriate actions and disregard for protocol.

Yet, Stephan was not solely a heartless brute, described by relatives as compassionate at times. He also exhibited symptoms of the 'the Mother Teresa syndrome', displaying a fervent dedication to his work. However, he often overstepped professional boundaries, such as personally calling families after a patient died, a task reserved for physicians. Interestingly, he never complained about witnessing patients' suffering.

Pattern

Gone are the sensational headlines proclaiming Stephan Letter as the post-World War II era's most notorious mass murderer, as the courtroom drama unfolds in February 2006 at the Kempten courthouse.

As Stephan, flanked by two guards, enters the hushed courtroom, a heavy silence descends, punctuated only by the creak of his shackles. His imposing figure, weighing 145 kilograms, is clad in a dark, impeccably tailored suit.

With the trial underway, Stephan delivers his statement, his voice devoid of emotion as he admits to bearing responsibility for the deaths of several patients. Yet, he vehemently denies the 28 murders attributed to him, claiming an inability to recall the exact number.

The revelation that Stephan cannot remember the precise number of victims elicits gasps of disbelief from the bereaved families seated in the gallery. Despite his remorseless demeanor, he offers a semblance of apology, attributing his actions to a tumultuous relationship with his now-ex-girlfriend.

As Stephan concludes his statement, the prosecutor lays bare the chilling facts. The police delved into a staggering eighty deaths occurring during the defendant's tenure. In their quest for evidence, forty-two bodies were exhumed, while the remaining thirty-eight had been consigned to cremation. Traces of the administered substances were unearthed in several of the exhumed remains.

Each victim, regardless of age or condition, met an unexpected demise. Significantly, these deaths unfolded during the defendant's solitary night shifts, offering ample opportunity for clandestine deeds with minimal oversight. The victims were not chosen based on their ailments; rather, the defendant's selection process was utterly random. Some had been under his care for days, while others were mere acquaintances of minutes. Their conditions ranged from critical illness to promising recovery. Astonishingly, a handful were not even within his purview, yet he brazenly trespassed into their rooms. Once his target was chosen, a methodical sequence ensued: first, a sedative to induce drowsiness, followed swiftly by a concoction of muscle relaxants, triggering a fatal paralysis of the respiratory system, culminating in suffocation within moments. The medications were injected directly into the intravenous line to minimize evidence. And so, he killed one sick person after another, as if it were assembly-line work. The intervals between the killings grew shorter over time, a common phenomenon among serial killers, indicative of a loss of control.

The defendant's professed motive of compassion is not taken seriously.

Defense's Plea

The courtroom buzzed with tension as the defense made their case, aiming to chip away at their client's culpability. They first criticized the investigators, arguing that they failed to explicitly inform their client after his arrest that he was only suspected of medication theft. But, according to the judge, they can hardly be blamed for this, because they themselves did not know that they were dealing with a serial killer.

Next, the defense targeted the lax medication control, highlighting how their client could clandestinely procure fifty vials of sedatives without raising suspicion. They also leveled accusations at the hospital, asserting that they had thrown their client, a recent nursing graduate, into the deep end by assigning him the care of critically ill patients. Seeking to widen the scope of the trial, the defense pressed for the inclusion of Stephan's girlfriend, currently institutionalized due to severe borderline personality disorder, citing a notion of a synergistic effect amplifying the combined pathology of two mentally compromised individuals. The lawyers also point out the devastating effect of Stephan's compulsive, neurotic mother during his childhood, an aspect that is also discussed in the final report of the psychological and psychiatric observation.

Stephan Letter, an above-average, intelligent man with an IQ of 121, is plagued by an extremely low sense of self-worth. The defendant's crimes unfolded over a period akin to a slowly evolving nuclear disaster. After being raised by his obsessive mother, he could no longer endure the pathological compulsion of his girlfriend, leading to an explosion of feelings of insignificance, personal and others' suffering. To avoid succumbing entirely to feelings of worthlessness, fantasies of omnipotence took hold, and he made the decision as to which patients should be put to sleep.

In the courtroom Stephan Letter's fate was sealed. Shackled and flanked by guards, he entered the courtroom amidst a deafening silence. Clad in a somber suit, his bulky frame loomed large as he stood before the judge.

Stephan Letter is deemed fully accountable for his actions. The role of his girlfriend remains outside the scope of the criminal proceedings, as it is the defendant standing trial, not anyone else. The judge aligns with the

187

prosecutor's demand and sentences him to life imprisonment for twelve counts of murder, fifteen counts of manslaughter, and one count of aiding suicide. Due to the gravity of his crimes, he will never be eligible for parole.

A year and a half later, during the appeal at the court in Karlsruhe, the verdict is reaffirmed.

Once again, this chapter underscores how wounds from one's youth can have far-reaching consequences. However, the perennial question persists: are these scars the sole reason behind one's criminal behavior, or is there also an inherent predisposition? The upcoming chapter delves into the story of an American nurse, whose actions, as far as can be traced, stem from traumatic childhood experiences. As a child, she endured unspeakable torment at the hands of her father.

17.

Black-outs

Terri Rachals, United States, 1985

Rapid Reaction

Between October 18 and November 26, 1985, a chilling wave swept through the cardiac intensive care unit of Phoebe Putney Memorial Hospital in Albany. Patients succumbed to cardiac arrest at an alarming rate, each one barely revived before the next fell victim. Hospital authorities acted swiftly, summoning law enforcement in early December. The Georgia Bureau of Investigation was tasked with unraveling the mystery that gripped the medical community.

As the hospital tightened its vigilance, preserving every piece of evidence, including used tubes and conducting meticulous laboratory tests, the cause remained elusive. An astute epidemiologist, who, delving into records, uncovered a startling revelation: in the year leading up to the epidemic, deaths averaged a mere zero to four per month. However, November painted a different picture, eleven sudden deaths, all occurring during the late shift under the watch of one nurse. What made this even more perplexing was the sudden cessation of cardiac arrests once the investigative team stepped in.

In early February, the cardiac ward was thrown into chaos when a patient suffered not one, but two consecutive heart attacks within a short span of time, despite being successfully resuscitated in between. The investigative team made a chilling discovery during the autopsy, an abnormally high level of a substance crucial for heart regulation, found both naturally in the body as can be assumed in medical form and plays a role in regulating the heart rate. Suspicion fell heavily on a particular nurse.

Terri Rachals, a dedicated nurse and mother, had spent the morning baking cookies with her beloved two-year-old son. Little did she know that her routine day would take a sinister turn. As she prepared to begin her evening shift, fate intervened in the form of two detectives waiting to question her. Bewildered and without a clue as to why she was being interrogated, Terri never even considered asking for legal representation. Instead, she requested the presence of the head nurse, desperate for support in the face of mounting accusations.

Detectives wasting no time in dropping their bombshell, claiming to possess evidence linking Terri to the sudden cardiac crises. As Terri was escorted out of the ward between the two detectives, her colleagues looked on in shock and disbelief, tears flowing freely. The once bustling cardiac unit was now shrouded in suspicion and sorrow, leaving everyone to wonder: could a trusted caregiver truly be capable of such sinister acts?

Trapped in Darkness

In the quaint village of Hopeful, nestled in the heart of Georgia, tragedy struck in 1964 as Terri's biological mother succumbed to a debilitating nervous breakdown. Left with no choice, she relinquished her two-year-old daughter, setting in motion a series of events that would forever alter Terri's life. Adopted by a childless couple in Albany, just fifty kilometers away, Terri's new beginnings held the promise of hope.

Albany, a vibrant African-American community, held its own charm with a square graced by the statue of legendary musician Ray Charles, born there in 1930. His timeless anthem *Georgia on My Mind* echoed through the streets, a testament to the city's rich cultural heritage. But for young Terri, the road ahead would be fraught with hardships.

Her adoptive parents, once stalwarts of the navy, now found themselves at different junctures in their careers. While the father had retired as an esteemed officer, the mother continued to serve in the civilian realm. Terri's days were spent in innocent play, nursing her mother in their make-believe hospital, a loving bond forged through imaginary injections and tender care. She was the picture of obedience, meticulously preparing her clothes for school, where she excelled academically.

Yet, tragedy struck when Terri's mother fell victim to a catastrophic brain hemorrhage, her life hanging by a thread. For days, Terri, just eleven years old, kept vigil by her mother's side, her father equally distraught. But in the end, they were left shattered, their world forever changed by the cruel hand of fate.

Did Terri's father seek refuge in his daughter's presence, both physically and emotionally, to fend off his own inner turmoil? Or had his troubled soul always teetered on the brink of darkness? One thing was certain, chaos reigned supreme within the walls of their home. While Terri struggled to focus on her studies, her father, lost in a haze of whiskey, laying sprawled on the couch, empty bottles littering the floor beside him. The silence was deafening, for Terri knew all too well the consequences of disturbing her father's slumber.

Until the age of sixteen, Terri was held captive by her father's demons and raped, living in fear of his unpredictable outbursts. A gun kept within arm's reach served as a grim reminder of the danger lurking within their household. And when Terri dared to oppose him, she found herself banished to the confines of the cellar, trapped in darkness and despair. It was only through sheer determination that she managed to break free, seeking sanctuary with relatives in the same city.

Amidst the turmoil of her upbringing, Terri found solace in caring for others. Her compassionate nature led her to pursue a career in nursing, a decision reinforced by her love for a physically challenged man whom she married after just one year together. With a swift immersion in the field of nursing, Terri embarked on a new chapter at Phoebe Putney Memorial Hospital in Georgia's medical landscape.

Sobbing Colleagues

Entering the highly specialized cardiac intensive care unit, the young woman navigated a world where heartbeats hung in the balance alongside neurological complexities. She favored the late shift, spanning from 3:00 PM to 11:00 PM, a schedule that allowed her to blend her devotion to her faith, harmonizing in the church choir on Sundays before visits to her husband's kin. Yet, whispers fluttered in the air, questioning whether she remained in touch with her father, a detail cloaked in mystery.

In appearance, the vibrant nurse bore a striking resemblance to the lead character of a beloved American TV series, *Murder She Wrote*, the iconic Jessica Fletcher portrayed by Angela Lansbury. Much like Fletcher, a widow immersed in unraveling mysteries within a fictitious coastal town, Terri exuded a warmth akin to the fictional sleuth. From the outset, she seamlessly meshed with her colleagues, her cheerful disposition a balm in the often-tense hospital environment. Engaged in team discussions and ever ready to swap shifts, Terri's dedication was unwavering. Three years into her tenure, motherhood graced her life, further enriching her days.

However, shadows danced amidst the flickering hospital lights as Terri confided in a coworker, revealing the hidden bruises of domestic violence staining her marriage. Her husband, juggling a small business alongside their shared parental duties, wielded violence as a twisted response to life's challenges. Though later offering glowing praise of her husband, Terri's initial disclosure lingered. As the plot thickened, the haunting specter of recurring domestic turmoil intertwined with the inexplicable string of cardiac arrests.

In the heart of a cardiac intensive care unit, where life and death dance in a delicate balance, the sudden surge of eleven cardiac arrests within a short span raises alarm bells. From a tender three-year-old to a soul nearing ninety, the victims spanned every age imaginable. And amidst tearful farewells from her colleagues, Terri finds herself flanked by detectives at the police station, where the weight of suspicion hangs heavy in the air. Did she deliberately administer unauthorized injections to these vulnerable patients? Initially resolute in her denial, Terri's resolve crumbles within the span of a half-hour interrogation, confessing to the unthinkable: administering potent medications meant to regulate heartbeats in their purest form, a stark deviation from standard protocol.

But as her words spill forth, there's a haunting detachment in her demeanor, as though the enormity of her admission eludes her grasp. Faced with the specter of imprisonment, she hints at thoughts of self-harm, triggering a flurry of psychiatric intervention and sedation. When offered admission to a psychiatric ward, she nods in silent assent, seeking solace in the embrace of her husband, who rushes to her side in a whirlwind of desperation.

Yet, as the fog of sedation lifts, Terri finds herself trapped in the cold confines of Dougherty County Jail, cut off from the outside world save for her attorney. Psychiatrists flood in, probing her mind until she's driven to desperate measures, etching 'Please leave me alone' on the walls. Recalling her first five days in confinement later, she can only recount three things: missing her son, the coarse texture of her blanket, and the monotony of her uniform dress, worn for three consecutive days. Initially charged with one count of murder, Terri's descent into the legal labyrinth begins.

Division

Newspapers blare the chilling moniker: *The Angel of Death from Phoebe*, as Terri finds herself behind bars. Yet, amidst the cacophony of accusations, a steady stream of support pours in, highlighting the stark divisions within the community. Despite the allegations, many rally behind Terri, steadfast in their belief in her innocence. According to one neighbor, she is the epitome of kindness, the last person one would suspect of malice.

As Terri prepares for her first court appearance, she follows her attorney's advice and retracts her earlier confession, citing coercion during interrogation. However, detectives adamantly maintain that she exhibited lucidity throughout their questioning. The lingering question persists: did

Terri truly grasp the gravity of her actions as she stood beside her patients' beds, moments before their heart monitors fell silent?

In the subsequent indictment, Terri faces charges of inflicting severe bodily harm twenty times and six counts of murder. What follows is a whirlwind legal battle, her trial unfolding at a remarkable pace, casting a harsh spotlight on the weight of the accusations against her.

In the courtroom drama unfolding, the question of guilt intertwines with the delicate intricacies of the defendant's mental state during the alleged crimes, setting the stage for a battle of psychiatric testimonies. On one side stands the defense's expert witness, attributing Terri's memory lapses during the incidents to a complex interplay of depression, her passive-aggressive nature, and dissociative amnesia stemming from years of unspeakable abuse at the hands of her father. This form of psychological self-defense, a complete black out if you want, akin to a protective cloak during moments of peril, can render individuals temporarily unaware of their actions, followed by a complete erasure of the traumatic event from memory.

This psychological phenomenon evokes shades of the trance-like state earlier described, where caregivers might find themselves lost in the emotional turmoil of their patients' suffering. Yet, here, it takes on a different hue, blending with a sense of infatuation amidst the turmoil. Dissociative amnesia, however, serves as a desperate survival tactic, shielding the mind from the unbearable weight of reality.

Opposing this narrative is the prosecution's psychiatric expert, vehement in his dissent, though his diagnosis offers no solace. He paints a portrait of Terri haunted by an abyss of self-loathing, a result of the harrowing abuse she endured, an unfortunate reality now beyond dispute. Unable to bear her own reflection due to overwhelming shame, she seeks to assert control over her tumultuous existence through the most chilling means - wielding power over life and death itself.

In addition, he finds no evidence that Terri's mind had temporarily slipped from reality. The defendant was fully cognizant of her actions when she administered the fatal injections to her victims. How else could she have confessed to the murders?

The mere fact that Terri was present near the victims during the cardiac arrests is deemed as circumstantial evidence.

According to the jury, the woman is deemed mentally disturbed but partly accountable, as the testimony of the prosecution's psychiatric expert is deemed the most credible. The jury absolves Terri of all murder charges and nearly all charges of severe bodily harm. However, she is found guilty of administering a lethal injection to an 89-year-old patient once. Terri claims that this patient had begged her to end his suffering. As the man's condition deteriorated due to severe thrombosis, which had already necessitated the amputation of his legs, the doctor prescribed plasma. Terri obtained a bag of plasma from the lab and clandestinely added a fatal dose of medication to it before connecting it to the IV line. When the man's heart rate plummeted, Terri promptly alerted a doctor. Although the patient was successfully resuscitated, he succumbed thirteen days later.

Terri Rachals is sentenced to seventeen years in a women's prison, along with an additional three years of probation. The higher court subsequently upholds her sentence.

Behind Bars

Other than Chapter 7's brief glimpse into Kath and Gwen's prison time, we know little about what happens to the convicts. But thanks to the correspondence between Terri Rachals and journalist Jennifer Furio for her book *Letters from Prison, Voices of Women Murderers*, published in 2001, their world opens up a little.

Jennifer Furio's unexpected request for Terri to contribute catches her off guard, particularly as she navigates a world where former friends have abandoned her, fostering a sense of distrust. Terri's sole focus remains protecting her son and husband from further harm. However, after studying the author's previous works, Terri reluctantly agrees to Jennifer's proposal, hoping to offer solace to fellow survivors of sexual abuse.

Over time, their correspondence becomes a lifeline for Terri, offering a semblance of connection in the bleakness of incarceration. She opens up about her efforts to navigate prison life, seeking to comprehend the events that led to her crimes through years of therapy. Terri's therapist helps her unearth the roots of her actions in her troubled past. These therapy sessions also serve as a means of coping with the harsh realities of prison, especially during the lonely and interminable nights.

Alone with her thoughts, Terri feels a profound sense of loneliness and detachment from the outside world, as fragments of her childhood memories flit through her mind. She vividly recalls the moments she begged God to make her father stop, the bitterness when her prayers went unanswered, and the rage over her father's actions. Terri draws chilling parallels between domestic violence and prison life: once it was her father shouting at her, now it's the prison guards. The fear grips her as they conduct unannounced cell searches, reminiscent of the trepidation she felt as a schoolgirl walking home along the dusty path after getting off the school bus. Desperately trying to conceal her tears, she wishes she could vanish. Her heart aches for her family, especially around her son's birthday. When she was arrested, he was just two and a half years old; now he's a young man learning to shave. Despite the distance, she's grateful their bond remains strong. She wrote him countless letters, even when he couldn't read, and he kept them all. The strain of the legal ordeal took its toll on her marriage, but she and her husband remain friends. The breaking point came when the newspapers portrayed him as a helpless invalid, emphasizing her obsessive need to care for him. Despite his slight limp and unclear speech, he's independent and cares for himself and their child.

After nine years behind bars, Terri writes a letter to the family of the only victim for which she was convicted, offering her heartfelt apologies for the pain she caused but insisting she never harbored malicious intent. There's no response.

Four years later, Terri tries again. She expresses her heartfelt regret, wishing a million times she could turn back the clock. Despite her traumatic past, she takes full responsibility for her actions, acknowledging she should never have ended the life of their 89-year-old father, and she pleads for forgiveness. This time, the family responds, accepting her remorse with gratitude. They hope the remaining years in prison will be less burdensome for her. In 2003, after exactly seventeen years, Terri Rachals is released.

The devastating impact of sexual abuse on its victims cannot be overstated, and Terri Rachals is not the only perpetrator who was a victim herself. Nearly thirty years ago, Donald Harvey murdered his first patient, also in the United States, but 750 kilometers north. He, too, was a victim of rape at a young age.

18.

Guinness Book of Records

Donald Harvey, United States, 1987

Ceremony

Draped in a somber black robe, its fabric clinging to his slender frame, he arranges the table with a macabre elegance, shrouding it in dark cloths. A skull, its top crudely sawed off, is positioned meticulously at the center of an antique bowl. Great that they didn't notice that he took that skull from the morgue. As the candle within the hollow cranium flickers to life and the pungent scent of incense fills the air, the ritual commences.

He now opens a book with magical texts and secures a sterile surgical mask over his face, obscuring his features. Then, in a hushed tone, he invokes the spirit of Duncan, a fellow disciple he met within the sinister depths of a satanic coven, the only confidant privy to his darkest confessions.

One by one, he lifts the trophies of his gruesome deeds above the makeshift altar: a half-crumbled cookie, a handful of worn socks, a tattered blanket, and a lock of hair, singed and withered by the heat of the flame. And then come the vessels containing his vile offerings of spit and blood, completing the ghastly tableau.

In the eerie silence, he whispers the names of the unsuspecting patients who will fall under his malevolent care that fateful night, his breath hitching with anticipation for a sign from his spectral ally. Only when the candle hesitantly flickers at the utterance of the third name does he know that his friend has answered his call.

The above information is only available to us because Donald Harvey's lawyer William Wahlen, with the consent and even at the request of his client, wrote a book about him so that healthcare workers with similar tendencies can be stopped in a timely manner. Donald's willingness is moving after he was convicted in 1987 of 36 murders and one manslaughter of unsuspecting patients.

Breeding Ground

In the bleak landscape of a small Ohio town in 1952, Donald Harvey's entry into the world was marked not by warmth and security, but by the shadow of turmoil. His mother, a mere seventeen years old and already haunted by her own demons, succumbed to postpartum depression after his birth, while his father, a distant figure consumed by work, was seldom present to offer solace.

At the tender age of two, Donald was stricken with convulsions during a bout of flu, further straining his family's fragile stability. As if scripted by fate, his mother welcomed two more children into the world in quick succession, each birth plunging her deeper into the abyss of despair.

Raised in the oppressive confines of a dilapidated home, young Donald's world was one of dampness and desolation, tattered curtains serving as a metaphor for the frayed edges of his fractured childhood.

By the time he reached the age of three, his parents' marriage dissolved, leaving him adrift in a sea of familial discord. His father's sporadic visits provided little comfort, and a tragic accident, where Donald fell from his father's truck, cast a dark shadow over his already troubled existence.

Despite the occasional respite provided by his maternal grandparents, Donald's role as the eldest sibling thrust him into a caretaker's role from an early age. His desperate act of defiance, the brutal dismemberment of a forbidden pet chick, hinted at the darkness lurking within his young soul.

At school, his fellow students think he is too girly and they call him 'sissy' or 'mother's boy'. And as if the misery wasn't great enough, he was regularly sexually abused by a neighbor and an uncle from the age of four. He endured this offense, during which he was regularly tied up, until he was ten years old. From that age until he was eighteen, Donald, yearning for any form of attention, took the initiative to contact his rapists. There is so little money coming in at home that the boy has to work part-time in a factory while still in high school. He also takes care of his grandmother, who is bedridden. He steals some money here and there and attends meetings of a neo-Nazi group because he adores Hitler. When Donald turns out to be homosexual, his relationship with his parents deteriorates. After graduating from high school, he moved to live on his own at the age of seventeen and worked as a ward assistant in a Catholic hospital run by nuns in London, Kentucky. There he committed his first murder at the age of eighteen.

Euphoria

Donald is usually early for work. On the way to the nursing station, he admires his image in uniform in the stained-glass windows. Human Resources is satisfied with the new addition. His neat appearance, good manners and the knowledge with which he cares for the sick make an impression. Because Donald puts his best foot forward, he is given more responsibilities. For example, he is the only one in the department who is allowed to catheterize male patients, for which he works extra overtime and even shows up outside of duty hours. On a busy afternoon he has to change a patient who has soiled himself with feces. The confused man accidentally soils Donald's spotless uniform and then then his fuses blow up. He presses a plastic bag and a pillow on the patient's face until he suffocates.

Serial killers describe how a first murder in particular is experienced as an unsurpassable euphoria and Donald Harvey is no different. Once he realizes that the patient is dead, an overwhelming feeling of relaxation occurs. As if by magic, he is no longer the weakling in his eyes, but someone with authority. In his first three months in this hospital, he kills six patients, and in the following 21 months he kills another seven. And every time afterwards he feels good about himself because he has outsmarted everyone. Shortly after his employment, he starts a relationship with a man twice his age, a funeral director. Donald watches his friend embalm the bodies. However, the man not only abuses the deceased, but also uses their organs for occult practices. When the two have an argument and the relationship comes under strain, Donald kills his last four victims in this hospital. Once he and his friend break up, Donald is quite upset. He breaks into his neighbor's house and sets fire to his apartment. In the evening and at night he wanders the streets looking for casual sex. When he is caught with a minor and is interrogated by the police, he confesses to killing fifteen patients in the hospital. But he is not believed.

Ruthless

Driven by his father's urging, Donald enlists in the Air Force at the tender age of nineteen. Yet, his military journey is abruptly cut short. Within nine months, it is discovered that he is using cocaine and the gates of the barracks close behind him. Officially cited reasons for his discharge include behavioral problems, depression, and incompetence.

With no other option, he returns temporarily to living at home. But we can assume this was not a success, as during this period Donald overdosed on medication three times, spending ninety days in a psychiatric hospital, undergoing shock therapy. After being discharged he continues visiting a psychiatrist. Shortly after this is terminated, he drives his car off a mountain road, plunging into the depths below. He escapes with minor injuries. During the subsequent trial for the later murders, he vehemently denies all his suicide attempts.

His path veers through a labyrinth of instability, marked by fleeting employment in the healthcare sector. Yet, amidst this tumult, he secures a foothold in a military hospital in Cincinnati, Ohio. Behind the façade of his impeccable demeanor, Donald prowls the corridors, he murders seventeen patients.

No one suspects a thing. In fact, he receives three bonuses and two special thanks for his dedication. Three days after killing his fifteenth victim, his head nurse notes in Donald's evaluation report that he scores 'well' on six out of ten and 'quite acceptable' on the remaining four criteria. There is only one downside: his judgment is 'moderate'.

Whether he is transferred at his own request or involuntarily is unknown, but he has been assisting with autopsy in the pathological-anatomical department for eight years. Shortly after moving in with his new boyfriend Carl, Donald starts killing outside the hospital.

Donald's possessiveness knows no bounds as he strives to keep Carl within arm's reach. Resorting to insidious tactics, he administers small doses of arsenic to his food, forcing Carl to call in sick. But Donald's malevolence extends beyond the confines of their home.

In a sinister twist, he poisons individuals in Carl's social circle, clandestinely tainting the meals of three tenants renting one of Carls apartments. Consequence: two lives tragically lost, while the rest endure harrowing illness before pulling through. Next, Carl's father falls victim and succumbs to the toxin. Carl's mother also becomes a target, but she survives.

However, Donald's extermination spree is far from over. At a party, fueled by jealousy, he sabotages a friend's salmon salad with poison, resulting in widespread vomiting among the guests. Fuelled by envy, Donald attempts to teach a lesson to a female employee of Carl by infecting her with blood contaminated with hepatitis and the AIDS virus, obtained from the hospital where he worked. The woman requires hospitalization but manages to survive.

As suspicions begin to mount, Carl realizes he must flee. Unable to afford the apartment rent alone, Donald retreats to living in a caravan.

While the full extent of Donald's atrocities remains unknown, he is ultimately caught during a routine check at the military hospital for an entirely different reason. A pistol, stolen medical books, syringes, and a tissue sample are discovered in his bag, after which he is asked to 'resign'.

The Scent of Almonds

In the summer of 1986, Donald secures a position at a nursing home in Cincinnati without his credentials being thoroughly checked. The facility, catering to elderly, terminally ill patients, where doctors here are perpetually overworked, routinely signing death certificates without scrutiny, a perfect fit for Donald's malevolent intentions.

Within months of his arrival, murmurs begin to circulate about an alarming increase in mortality rates. It's a keen-eyed pathologist who first detects a faint, bitter almond odor emanating from the stomach contents of a motor accident victim, and he suspects cyanide poisoning. Yet, emboldened by his string of successful murders, Donald feels untouchable and refuses to cease his deadly activities.

Despite the brave efforts of whistleblowers, who face dismissal and intimidation, it takes a courageous journalist's exposé on a local radio station to shed light on the suspicious deaths.

Whereupon one of the journalists investigates himself and eventually sends a message into the air about the number of suspicious deaths.

Finally, an official investigation is launched, revealing cyanide in the stomachs of several deceased patients. It later emerges that during Donald's thirteen-month tenure at the facility, he claimed the lives of twenty-four innocent victims. His actions also have far-reaching consequences for numerous higher-ups who ignored whistleblowers' warnings.

Seventy

Following an exhaustive investigation, 172 potential victims emerge from the shadows of three hospitals, casting a dark cloud of suspicion over Donald. Sensing the tightening noose, he swiftly withdraws his savings, vehemently denying any involvement in a televised interview. Yet, beneath his veneer of innocence, he carries a vial of cyanide at all times, a chilling insurance policy for his own escape.

During his initial police interrogation, Donald confesses to one murder but remains tight-lipped about the rest. Managing to pass a lie detector test by reading a book on how to beat it. Assigned lawyer William Wahlen finds him in a state of utter despair: wide-eyed and huddled in a corner of his cell like a frightened animal. When asked if he has killed more patients, Donald immediately confesses to seventy.

Throughout the trial, Donald maintains his facade of innocence, but as damning evidence mounts, he finally buckles, admitting to his role in fifty-four deaths. Though the full extent of his crimes remains elusive, he is convicted on thirty-six counts of murder and one of manslaughter.

Amidst the courtroom drama, a unique bond forms between Donald and his defender, setting the stage for William Wahlen's later account in *Defending Donald Harvey, The Case of the Most Notorious Angel-of-Death Serial Killer* (2005). The lawyer is astounded by his client's astonishingly precise recollection of events.

To His Liking

With a chilling precision, Donald vividly recounts the horrors he unleashed within the walls of three healthcare facilities over nearly two decades, sparing only eleven victims from his detailed recollection. The murders committed beyond the hospital's confines remain a silent shadow.

The details of his first murder are etched in chilling clarity. Though the patient may have accidentally suffocated, Donald finds this method to his liking, as he proceeds to kill five more in a similar manner. In one instance, the crime takes a slightly different turn: a dying man, nearing exhaustion, would have naturally passed away if not for the nurse's intervention, who inadvertently caused him to suffocate by turning him onto his stomach.

In the aftermath of his initial murder, Donald's brutality escalates even more. Tasked with a routine procedure on a frail, resistant patient, he takes it upon himself to assert dominance, resulting in the man's untimely demise from sheer excitement.

This pattern of lethal aggression repeats itself, culminating in a chilling encounter with a trembling, bewildered patient. Fuelled by rage, Donald plots his vengeance, culminating in a calculated act of violence, a grotesque insertion of an oversized catheter, leaving the man in a coma, his life slipping away over four agonizing days.

In his dark repertoire of crimes, this perpetrator wielded a chilling array of methods, employing roughly five different techniques with callous efficiency. Much like his murders outside the hospital, he turned to poison, cyanide and arsenic, readily available in his caravan, to dispatch twenty-one victims. The poison was cunningly mixed into pudding or injected directly into their IV tubing or gastric tubes. Shockingly, in a macabre twist, he even administered the lethal substance into someone's testicles.

But Donald's depravity didn't stop there. With a sinister cunning, he tampered with oxygen equipment, denying five patients the vital air they needed, a nefarious act that went undetected amidst the chaos of the hospital wards. Three unfortunate souls met their demise through lethal injections: the first, an overdose of a blood-thinning agent, leading to fatal bleeding during surgery, the true cause concealed forever. The other two were victims of opioid overdoses.

When conventional means were lacking, Donald's twisted creativity knew no bounds. In four instances, he injected a chilling amount of air into a patient's vein, a cruel and silent killer. Or, on a chillingly calculated day, he allowed solvent meant for adhesive residue to seep into the lungs of two patients via their breathing tubes, sealing their fates with lethal efficiency.

Complaint

In the chilling chronicles of his crimes, Donald's deeds are often shrouded in secrecy, but glimpses of his actions emerge in the most unexpected places. At his second and sixth heinous acts, a nun from the first hospital where he toils bears witness to his sinister endeavors. Silently, she gestures, pressing her index finger to her lips, a silent plea for secrecy that Donald obediently heeds.

As Donald recounts his dark deeds, a pattern of interruptions emerges, disrupting his deadly plans with at least five victims, forcing him to repeat his actions. With his 29th victim, he grapples with frustration, administering arsenic four times as the poisoned food repeatedly meets the hospital floor. In a twisted display of gratitude, the widow of his 26th victim hosts a lunch for the hospital staff, unaware of the sinister undercurrents.

Despite his calculated cruelty, traces of humanity flicker within Donald's cold facade. The end of his relationship with Carl marks the commencement of his 28th murder, a chilling testament to his emotional detachment. Then, with his 34th victim, a swift reaction to cyanide catches Donald off guard, prompting him to call for assistance. However, his plea falls on deaf ears as the patient, under a 'do not resuscitate' order, is left to face death alone, leaving Donald feeling slighted enough to lodge a complaint.

Amidst the darkness of his crimes, a fleeting moment of empathy too surfaces. Before claiming his 36th victim, Donald pauses, waiting for the patient's wife to visit áfter her vacation, because he doesn't want to spoil her holiday. I would say, a small act of mercy in the midst of unspeakable horror.

Indifferent

Throughout the trial, Donald seemed to revel in the attention, his demeanor surprisingly genial as he sat alert in the defendant's chair. It was hard for observers to reconcile this outward affability with the heinous crimes he was accused of. The psychiatric-psychological report is scrutinizing with rapt attention.

Described as an intelligent yet compulsive serial killer, Donald found satisfaction in preying upon the most vulnerable, those utterly dependent on him. The report painted a chilling picture of a man whose cunning evaded detection for far too long, all while retaining full accountability for his actions.

The report didn't shy away from highlighting the defendant's psychopathic traits, notably his unflinching gaze devoid of remorse during interrogation. The immeasurable suffering inflicted upon his victims seemed to leave him indifferent, the only remorse he exhibits is for being caught.

Despite the severity of the accusations against him, Donald displayed a surprising amount of pride, vehemently disputing any misattributed details presented by the prosecutor.

Although it may seem incongruous for a condemned man facing severe punishment to jest, Donald doesn't hesitate to inject humor into the proceedings. When one of the witnesses requests a glass of water, he ironically remarks that it would surely be undesirable for him to fill the glass. According to the report, Donald's humor isn't genuine but merely serves a theatrical purpose, momentarily drawing attention back to himself.

Even behind bars, Donald's aspirations didn't wane, as he requested a copy of the latest *Guinness Book of Records*, disappointed to find his name absent.

Donald's own explanation for his actions revealed a disturbing mindset, wherein he claimed to only act out when feeling unwell, viewing the taking of lives as a means to alleviate his own feelings of worthlessness. His escalating sense of power and control culminated in a belief that he held the roles of judge, jury, prosecutor, and even God all at once.

In the end, the court delivered its verdict, sentencing Donald to four consecutive life terms and imposing a hefty fine of $270,000.

For the families of his victims, the closure brought by the verdict offered little solace in the wake of their unimaginable loss. Donald's actions had irrevocably shattered countless lives, leaving behind a trail of devastation that would linger for years to come.

19.

The untouchable

Colin Norris, England, 2002

Stumbling Into Their Own Trap

In the courtroom nestled by the murmuring River Tyne in Newcastle, a hushed conversation passes between lawyer and client. Colin Norris, with a determined stride, steps into the spotlight. His advocate, with an air of unwavering confidence, dismisses the prosecution's feeble case, adamantly declaring the absence of any witness to Norris's alleged injections of insulin into patients. Why indeed would he be the one to draw suspicion? Within the walls of a hospital, a realm of public accessibility, one might question the singling out of Colin Norris. Could the unfortunate demise of the patients be simply attributed to the natural ebb and flow of their blood sugar levels? Yet, as the defense lauds Norris's supposed impeccable bedside manner, they inadvertently stumble into a pit of their own making. Little did they know, the prosecutor had tactfully withheld mention of Norris's less than savory conduct, opting not to influence the jury prematurely. The judge's response is swift and unequivocal: 'You are mistaken! The demeanor of the accused was far from polite!'

His Early Years

In the heart of Glasgow's St. Patrick district, amidst the clangor of industry, lies the humble beginning of Colin Norris. Born to young parents, his father a mere 21 and his mother even younger, Colin's childhood is marked by their absence as they toil away at their respective jobs: his father behind the wheel of a taxi, his mother tapping away as a typist. Left in the care of his maternal grandmother during their working hours, she becomes a steadfast presence in his life.

Colin grows up an only child, finding solace in the world of drama at his primary school and camaraderie within the ranks of the Boy Scouts. But beneath his jovial exterior lies a brewing storm. At the tender age of seven, his parents part ways, leaving Colin feeling abandoned by his father, who fades into the periphery of his life.

His mother, seeking a fresh start, moves in with her second husband, a burly builder with a young son of his own. They settle in a home just around the corner from Colin's grandmother, where he spends countless hours soaking in her love and wisdom.

Despite his lackluster academic performance in secondary school, Colin carves out a niche as the class clown, a phenomenon more common among healthcare serial killers, wielding his dry humor as a shield against the turmoil brewing within. Little do those around him know, behind the laughter lies a darkness waiting to be unleashed.

In the gritty tapestry of his upbringing, Colin's story begins with a moment of betrayal that sets the stage for a lifetime of turmoil. At seventeen, in a reckless act of defiance, he steals £20 from his grandfather's wallet on the eve of his grandmother's funeral, an act that severs already fragile familial ties. His father, incensed by the betrayal, cuts all contact, leaving Colin adrift in a sea of unresolved anger.

But Colin's vendetta doesn't end there. A year later, he demands £18,000 in retribution for the pain of his parents' divorce a decade earlier, further cementing his estrangement from his father.

As he navigates the tumultuous waters of adolescence, Colin grapples with his own sexuality, his preference for men, he confides in his mother, finding solace in her unwavering support.

Feeling positive, the lure of adventure beckons, and Colin sets his sights on a career in tourism and recreation, abandons his studies and finds himself immersed in the world of travel, booking exotic vacations for eager globetrotters.

Yet, it's during a fateful emergency first aid course that Colin's true calling reveals itself. Inspired by the prospect of making a tangible difference in people's lives, he sets his sights on a career in nursing, unaware of the dark path that lies ahead.

Authority Issues

In the industrial heartland of Dundee, Colin embarks on a tumultuous journey through a three-year nursing program. But his time there is marked by discord. Skipping classes becomes a habit, and he struggles academically, failing to stand out among his peers. Yet, it's his clashes with authority that truly define his experience.

At the slightest critique from his instructors, Colin's temper flares, leading to heated confrontations with his study mentor. He dismisses her as lacking in backbone, while she attributes his behavior to arrogance and stubbornness.

During his practical training, Colin's troubles follow him. Assigned to Ward 11 at Ninewells Hospital in the same town, where diabetic patients are common, his disdain for authority manifests in disturbing ways. When faced with a simple task like changing a patient's bedding after an accident, Colin refuses, a clear display of his disregard for protocol.

His frustrations only deepen during his second placement at Ward 7 of the local Royal Victoria Hospital. Expecting excitement in an emergency setting, Colin finds himself relegated to a geriatric ward, further fueling his resentment and paving the way for darker days ahead.

With a chip on his shoulder and a vocal aversion to the elderly, Colin's discontent reverberates through the halls of Riverside Victoria Hospital.

Despite management's attempts to accommodate him, relocating him to a setting with even more senior patients, Colin's dissatisfaction only deepens. His abrupt departure after a mere three days speaks volumes, yet surprisingly, the university lets him slip through their fingers without consequence.

During his nursing education, Colin attends a lecture that chronicles the case of Jessie McT., a nurse from his hometown of Glasgow, acquitted on appeal due to procedural errors. She had been sentenced to life in 1975 for the murder of one patient and four counts of attempted murder by insulin overdose, suspected of having 22 victims. Oddly, during his own trial, Colin claims not to remember this lecture, despite strikingly similar actions a year later.

At 25, armed with his nursing diploma, Colin ventures south to Leeds General Infirmary in October 2001, seeking a fresh start. His belongings packed in a van, he embarks on the journey, unaware of the tumultuous years that lie ahead.

Settling in Leeds, Colin enters into a series of living arrangements with different male partners, each harboring secrets that will eventually unravel during his trial, exposing the sinister truth lurking behind his facade of normalcy.

Clairvoyant

In the corridors of his first post-graduate hospital, despite the ongoing clashes during his orientation, he secures a permanent position in the orthopedic department. Where much like during his internship, the majority of patients under his care are elderly. Finding solace in the darkness outside, sneaking out through the fire exit for a quiet cigarette during the long night shifts.

But it's in the quiet hours before dawn that tragedy strikes. A patient, only a week removed from hip surgery, is discovered in a dire state, gasping for air, her consciousness slipping away. Yet days earlier she had been sitting upright in bed, engaging in animated conversation with her roommates over tea and scones.

As the medical team rushes to her aid, the shocking truth emerges: her blood sugar levels are dangerously low, an anomaly for a non-diabetic patient. Yet, further investigation uncovers a disturbing revelation, her bloodstream is saturated with insulin, far beyond what could be attributed to human error. The implications are grim: irreversible brain damage and a tragic demise.

As detectives delve into the situation, they uncover four more elderly women in the past six months whose conditions deteriorated suddenly. Like the woman enjoying tea and scones, they were all challenging, demanding, and incontinent, yet they were not diabetic.

In the silent depths of the night, the ward bears witness to a series of tragedies. Five months into his tenure, Colin experiences his first encounter with death, a fragile 90-year-old woman, her leg fractured, barely clinging to consciousness when discovered late in the evening, long after Colin has left his post. Miraculously, she manages to pull through.

But the specter of mortality lingers, haunting the ward with its presence. Six weeks later, an 80-year-old heart patient is found in a similar state, her life slipping away just minutes after Colin's departure in the morning light.

Four weeks pass, and Colin's night shift takes a grim turn as he stumbles upon an 88-year-old woman, her body still and unresponsive. Within hours, she succumbs to the silent call of death.

Despite the growing toll, Colin is discreetly relocated to St. James's Hospital, where the darkness of night reveals yet another victim, a 79-year-old woman, found in a diabetic coma. Colin's unnerving stillness by her bedside raises suspicions, compounded by the discovery of an empty insulin stock.

Yet, amidst the veil of tragedy, no alarms are raised. The woman breathes her last on her birthday, her passing unnoticed. Strikingly enough, that when the Colin finds her, he remains standing next to her bed like a pillar of salt, as if it does not concern him as the responsible nurse. A colleague also discovers that the stock of insulin in the refrigerator has run out.

In the meticulous scrutiny of nursing reports, a sinister prophecy emerges from the shadows of nurse Colin's words. An hour before the tragic demise of the woman who savored her tea ceremony, Colin's unsettling premonition unfolded in a conversation with a colleague. 'There's something not right about her', he confided, his apprehension shrouded in vague unease. 'I bet you, these elderly ones always slip away during my shift. I give her until quarter past five,' words laden with an eerie certainty. His colleague, perplexed, furrowed her brow.

As they stood beside the bed of the struggling, unconscious patient, Colin's demeanor shifted to one of triumph. With a tap of his watch, he declared, 'There you go, just as I said'.

The detectives catch the faint scent of a trail, leading them deeper into the shadows of suspicion. With each discovery of an unconscious patient, Colin Norris's presence looms ominously. Delving into the annals of medical records, experts meticulously dissect all 72 deaths under Colin's watchful eye. Eighteen cases emerge as focal points, weaving a tangled web of suspicion around nurse Colin's involvement in the tragic demise of five vulnerable women.

Holiday Pictures

Amidst the somber corridors of suspicion, a self-assured figure perches at the desk. It's a common trait among healthcare serial offenders to don an air of arrogance when the spotlight of suspicion shines upon them. When confronted with his potential involvement, Colin snaps back at the detectives, his tone dripping with disdain, 'How could you even think such a thing?'

As snapshots of the victims are laid before him, Colin nonchalantly claims recognition of only one, dismissing the others as insignificant. Yet, these were the very souls he tended to day in and day out. To him, their deaths were nothing more than unfortunate coincidences, mere casualties of fate.

The lead investigator recalls Colin Norris's demeanor with a mix of disgust and disbelief. Rather than exhibiting any semblance of remorse or guilt, Colin's demeanor is one of defiance. He adamantly denies any wrongdoing, his arrogance shielding him from the weight of the accusations. At times, he even refuses to engage, storming out of interrogations in a fit of rage, only to return once his temper has cooled.

Unfortunately, due to a lack of formal charges, the detectives are forced to release him for the time being, suspended by his employer, who fears the worst. Packing his belongings back into the van and returning to Glasgow. Almost as if to mock the detectives, he boards a plane to a sunny destination and upon his return, strolling through the city's streets, bronzed from his vacation, gleefully showing his holiday photos.

While the suspect basks in the sun, detectives gather 7,000 statements, seizing 3,000 pieces of evidence, including duty rosters, pharmacy order forms, nursing reports, and patient records. Unexpectedly a revelation emerges: on days when Colin called in sick or had to attend training at Leeds General Infirmary, he worked four shifts at two other hospitals through a temp agency.

The data paints a different picture from the one the nurse portrays of himself. Allegedly refusing to empty the urine collection bag of a gravely ill man, insisting he could walk himself, pointing to the toilet down the hall. While attempting to get out of bed, the patient falls, resulting in serious injury.

Other patients testify that when they asked for help, the nurse either turned away or, in the worst cases, verbally abused them.

In October 2005, almost three years after his initial interrogation, Colin Norris is finally formally charged with four counts of murder and one count of attempted murder, and he is apprehended.

Grandma's Shadow

As the trial unfolds in October 2007, stretching over nineteen grueling weeks, Colin's demeanor remains unyielding. Approaching the courthouse with an aura of defiance, he startles a photographer with an unexpected blow, momentarily throwing off the composure of the slender nurse with his oversized glasses.

Yet, once settled in the defendant's seat, Colin's confidence returns in full force. With each assertion of innocence, he challenges the prosecutor's case, standing firm and speaking out against every accusation. His upright posture and smug expression betray an unwavering belief in his own righteousness, as he confidently corrects expert testimonies to fit his narrative.

Acknowledging his training on insulin's effects during his initial internship, Colin also confesses to his aversion to caring for geriatric patients, an admission that hints at deeper discomfort. He reluctantly admits his reluctance to bathe elderly women, a task reminiscent of his own grandmother's age, with a candid acknowledgment of the distressing scent that accompanied such duties. And as for his seemingly callous remarks about predicting death times, Colin dismisses them as mere gallows humor, a coping mechanism common among those entrenched in the somber realities of hospital life.

A former partner of the suspect testifies how Colin avidly following the hospital TV series *Holby City*, in which one of the episodes revealed a doctor to be a serial killer. Where also nurse Kelly in the series murdered a patient with morphine. Already suspected, Colin boasted about the similarities between the suspicions and developments in the series and what was happening to him.

A second former lover reveals that the neighbor saw Colin injecting their three rabbits with a syringe, who were shortly thereafter buried. When asked for an explanation, Colin swore he had given the rabbits vitamins. Only later did he admit it was insulin.

Apparently, no one lasted long with Colin, as another partner testifies that Colin also gave the cat an injection. When the relationship had apparently cooled, this partner reported Colin to the police. However, Colin claimed that the cat had died after running into a wall.

But what fueled Colin's heinous acts? A forensic psychiatrist peered into the abyss of his mind, revealing a disturbing desire to wield power and control. Each murder, a twisted assertion of dominance over those who dared cross his path, fueled by a narcissistic thirst for superiority.

A psychologist sees a craving for power in the behavior of the suspect. Competition with superiors may have also played a role. Because doctors didn't suspect anything, the nurse's ego grew. This feeling was further reinforced when doctors issued a natural death certificate.

Premeditation

In the hushed courtroom, the judge's words echoed like a solemn verdict from the depths of justice's conscience. According to the judge, it remains a matter of guessing the motive. He asks the jury to consider why the suspect was able to so accurately predict the death of the victim that started the whole case. The answer, elusive yet damning, emerged in the jury's resolute decision: Colin stood convicted by an overwhelming majority, eleven to one.

His facade of disbelief crumbling, his eyes locking with his lawyer's in a silent plea for reprieve from the merciless truth. But there was no escape from the harsh reality that awaited him. He receives four life sentences plus twenty years for the four murders: the 80-year-old woman, the 88-year-old woman, the 79-year-old lady, and the 86-year-old patient who enjoyed her tea. He is also convicted of attempted murder of the 90-year-old woman.

In the intricate tapestry of circumstantial evidence, the judge discerned a chilling narrative of premeditation. Only a heart steeped in malevolence could have orchestrated the injection of a lethal dose of insulin, sealing the fate of innocent lives.

Colin looks at his lawyer in disbelief. He had not taken a conviction into account at all.

This verdict, however, was a departure from the norm. Unlike typical trials where concrete evidence is the linchpin of conviction, the complexities of proving serial murders within the healthcare realm demanded a closer examination.

Suspects usually deny, and guilt is not always easy to establish. One-third are acquitted, sometimes on appeal, sometimes much later, years after a conviction. The first reason for this is that the alleged crimes occur within a caregiver relationship, nullifying the perpetrator-victim contact as evidence. Secondly, the presence of a drug in the victim's body does not rule out that the substance was not already produced by the body itself during resuscitation or administered accidentally in the wrong dose. Thirdly, an eyewitness report contributes evidentially only when the same witness has seen the defendant draw injection fluid from a specific ampule and then observed them administer the substance.

May 2024: due to doubts by some as to Colin Norris's guilt, his case is being reviewed by the Criminal Cases Review Commission who referred the case back to the Court of Appeal.

20.

The man who heard voices

Kurt Dobbelaere, Belgium, 2007

Candid Snapshots

Belgium, a country where even the most solemn of trials in the esteemed Court of Assizes carries an air of casualness unlike anywhere else. March 26, 2010, a day like any other in the bustling legal arena, yet devoid of the usual security checks at the entrance. Amidst the anticipation of jurors and court officials, a peculiar scene unfolds, a staff member, moonlighting as a renowned crime author, discreetly captures candid snapshots of the arriving audience. Not even the incessant ringing of mobile phones manages to disrupt the pre-trial buzz.

In the heart of the courtroom, two impeccably attired female attorneys adorn themselves in the traditional legal garb, their only companion a solitary can of diet cola. The audience, a diverse mix of onlookers, fills the room to the brim, with reserved seating at the forefront for grieving relatives and scattered family members of the accused. Tension hangs thick in the air, fueled by the gravity of the charges, four counts of murder and one of attempted murder.

As the defendant, a stooped figure with a pallid, weathered countenance, is escorted into the room, the stark reality of the situation sets in. At just forty-six, he bears the weariness of a man twice his age. For twenty-three long months since his apprehension, he has clung to the audacious claim of executing his actions under the sinister influence of his deceased mother. However, before the trial even commences, he shatters the façade with a startling admission: the voices he claimed to have obeyed were nothing but figments of his imagination.

Whispers of Suspicion

It was a seemingly routine day on August 30, 2007, when a 93-year-old resident of retirement home Privilege was admitted to the renowned academic hospital Sint-Lucas in Ghent. Initial concerns pointed to a minor cerebral hemorrhage, but the attending physician couldn't shake off the nagging doubts surrounding the case. Anomalies surfaced, an abnormally low blood sugar level and three inexplicable puncture wounds on the elderly woman's thigh.

Dr. X, troubled by the inconsistencies, reached out to the nursing home's care coordinator, Kurt Dobbelaere, seeking clarification on a crucial detail: was the patient diabetic? Kurt's response, a firm denial, only deepened the physician's suspicions. Doubt lingered, prompting a second call from the doctor.

'Are you absolutely certain?'

Kurt remained resolute. He discovered the woman in a semi-comatose state, yet her blood sugar levels were within the normal range. 'But' according to him 'She had lost the will to live'. Finding her in the morning, gasping for breath, she had said she wanted to die.

Days passed, and the unsettling puzzle took a darker turn. Kurt's subsequent revelation to the doctor, the discovery of four empty insulin ampoules tucked away in the woman's medication box, sent shockwaves through the medical team. The daughter, however, vehemently denied any suicidal tendencies in her mother, insisting that the medication box had been empty prior.

Despite the physicians' best efforts, the patient's condition deteriorated, ultimately leading to her demise thirteen agonizing days later. Fueled by a daughter's intuition and a growing sense of unease, suspicions blossomed into a full-blown investigation. The daughter's call to the authorities set in motion a chain of events that would unravel a web of deceit and betrayal lurking within the halls of Retirement home Privilege.

Months later, the same hospital bore witness to yet another harrowing ordeal. An 82-year-old resident, also from Retirement home Privilege, lay comatose, her life hanging by a thread. The similarities to the previous case were too striking to ignore. Dr. X, haunted by past shadows, knew instinctively that something sinister lurked beneath the surface.

Whispers of suspicion echoed through the corridors of the hospital, reaching the ears of law enforcement. The intricate tapestry of lies and deception unraveled further as the case landed in the hands of the federal judicial police.

Theft

In contrast to most other serial killers, Kurt Dobbelaere did not have a traumatized childhood. And it was in the quaint provincial town of Eeklo, nestled just 35 kilometers northwest of Ghent, a seemingly unremarkable tale unfolds. It is here, in 1964, that Kurt Dobbelaere enters the world as the firstborn in a devout Catholic household. A nurturing environment, by all outward appearances, yet beneath the surface, seeds of discontent begin to take root in young Kurt's heart.

Raised under the watchful eye of a dominating mother who presided over a home-based hairdressing salon. His father, a mere shadow in the background, toiled away in shift work, while Kurt and his younger brother navigated the complexities of childhood.

As the years passed, whispers of anomalies echoed through Kurt's surroundings. Money went missing, Belgian francs vanished from his brother's pockets, a friend's purse grew lighter, and even a customer's bills disappeared from the depths of a handbag. Kurt's mother, quick to shield her son from scrutiny, attributed the incidents to mere accidents, a narrative that fractured trust within the family's sanctum.

Locked cabinets became the norm, and Kurt, denied the autonomy of his own house key until his thirtieth year, bore witness to the erosion of familial bonds. Yet, amidst the turmoil, Kurt's aspirations took shape. Being an average student at school. Arriving late once, he lied that his grandmother had died.

Denied the path of a hairdresser by his mother's decree, he embarked on a tumultuous journey through various vocations, from horticulture to a fleeting dalliance with teaching.

But it was Kurt's ventures into matters of the heart that truly tested his resolve. Two relationships, each met with disapproval from his formidable matriarch, crumbled under the weight of her disdain. And as fate would have it, chronic asthma spared Kurt from the rigors of military service, leading him down an unexpected path into the realm of nursing.

Sad Reputation

In the annals of Kurt Dobbelaere's life, a tapestry of contradictions weaves a tale of perplexing complexity. Kurt's early years appeared unremarkable. His teachers remember him as a diligent student, yet classmates struggled to define his essence.

Upon earning his nursing diploma in 1987, Kurt embarked on a journey in healthcare. From the intense atmosphere of a hospital's intensive care unit to the gentle embrace of a nursing home, and finally, to the labyrinthine halls of a psychiatric center, Kurt's career path seemed diverse yet fraught with underlying tensions.

Amidst his professional endeavors, Kurt's personal life bore witness to a tempest of emotions. His courtship with Martine, his future wife, was marred by the harshness of Kurt's mother, driving Martine to tears on numerous occasions.

Their path to marital bliss took an unconventional turn as they ventured into homeownership, legally bound but geographically apart until their eventual church wedding. However, the joy of parenthood in 1996 was clouded by Kurt's resurgence into his old habits, the misappropriation of funds, this time from a cousin's wallet.

The summer of 1998 marked a pivotal moment as Kurt transitioned into running his own bustling practice as a private home nurse, to care for his sick mother, who is diagnosed with colon and liver cancer until her death at the age of 55 a year later. One of his other patients spots two of her missing rings in a jeweler's shop window. Kurt denies any involvement, but he is nevertheless sentenced to five years' probation for breach of trust, fraud, and forgery to the detriment of thirteen patients, and is required to undergo psychiatric treatment. Complying only if his wife accompanies him to the sessions, where, according to her, he barely speaks. The psychiatrist diagnoses him as manic-depressive and prescribes antidepressants. Once again, Martine ensures he takes his pills. Kurt embezzles 15,000 francs as treasurer from his own soccer club.

Burning Question

Despite a suspended sentence hanging over him like a dark cloud, as a nurse he continued his care for the sick, seamlessly transitioning through various nursing homes over the years. It wasn't until his employment at Privilege in October 2006 that his murky past caught up with him, culminating in his arrest by the end of 2007.

The burning question remains: how did he manage to slip through the cracks, securing employment at three subsequent nursing homes despite his tainted record? The answer lies in a web of deception, spun with calculated precision. Presenting himself to hiring committees with a carefully crafted tale of financial misfortune at his previous workplace, he managed to evade scrutiny, his words taken at face value without a single reference checked.

However, a pattern of unsettling behavior soon emerged, painting a disturbing portrait of a man veiled in deceit. Once hailed for his zeal and dedication, his colleagues soon grew wary as the veneer of charm gave way to a darker reality. Whispers of fear rippled through the corridors, as accusations of extortion, stalking, and intimidation tainted his reputation. Staff members are fearful and resign. In hindsight, Kurt is described as a power-hungry, deceitful smooth talker who never meets your gaze. In all facilities, money and belongings disappear, and Kurt is accused of extortion, stalking, unwanted advances, and sexual intimidation. A manipulative figure weaving a web of lies and deceit, leaving behind a trail of shattered trust and unanswered questions. In the eyes of those who knew him best, he was a shadowy figure, never meeting their gaze, his actions betraying the very essence of his being.

Family Enterprise

Kurt had a knack for turning flames into profit. While working at the psychiatric center, a patient's bathroom mysteriously caught fire, leaving investigators puzzled. Years later, Kurt himself caused a kitchen fire at his home, blaming it on a crumb vacuum and pocketing a hefty insurance payout.

Retirement home Privilege, where Kurt later worked, was a family-run business, a common setup in Belgium. Managed by a sister and brother without medical backgrounds, a facility housing 56 residents in an aging building in Ghent. Their father was on the board alongside representatives from the medical field, while their mother handled catering duties.

Even here, Kurt didn't hesitate to exploit a fire incident for personal gain. After a resident's epileptic seizure resulted in flames erupting from a pillow, Kurt feigned injury while extinguishing the fire and demanded a hefty compensation from the resident.

By the time of Kurt's arrest, he had been plagued by insomnia for months. Known for his excessive work ethic, he would even demand entering the retirement home in the early hours of the morning. Meanwhile, a strange incident occurred at his home, his garage inexplicably flooded. When his wife, still reeling from the recent kitchen fire and insurance matters, refused to call the insurance company, Kurt's temper flared.

Completely Uprooted

Just three days after returning from a period of absence marked by the loss of his father-in-law, Kurt embarked on a chilling path of deceit and manipulation. Injecting an 85-year-old woman, confused and debilitated by age, with a lethal dose of insulin, Kurt plunged into the depths of depravity. Despite the woman being found in a state of sub comatose, Kurt brazenly falsified records, noting her as devoid of signs of death while she still clung to life.

During interrogation, Kurt spun a tale of maternal coercion, claiming his mother had directed him to end the woman's life, an act he alleged was rewarded with a kiss on his brow. Undeterred by the horrors of his first crime, Kurt repeated his deadly charade the following day, targeting an 88-year-old man suffering from Parkinson's disease. Half an hour after administering the injection, he offered washing the man himself, a task outside his duties as a care coordinator. Unaware of the deliberate attempt on the man's life, the family also opted for a wait-and-see approach. After the man's death later that day, his daughter found a wooden cross in his hands. Given his symptoms, the Parkinson's patient could not have picked it up himself. As the man succumbed to the insulin, Kurt's eerie inquiry about cremation dates hinted at a deeper darkness lurking within.

Five days later, Kurt injected a lethal dose into a 93-year-old resident, the same woman who had been noted by the admitting physician for three puncture wounds on her thigh. Chilling whispers filled the courtroom as a paramedic recounted hearing a nursing assistant's eerie claim in the elevator that the nursing home was cursed, with this resident being the third in a week to require urgent medical intervention. The forensic pathologist's testimony painted a grim picture of brain damage from oxygen and sugar deprivation, consistent with insulin overdose, further deepening the macabre narrative.

The next day, Kurt targeted a demented 86-year-old woman, another of his victims, with a fatal injection between six and six-thirty in the morning. As she failed to awaken, the attending physician suspected a minor stroke, yet no treatment was initiated, leading to her passing the following day.

Amidst these horrors, Kurt's abrupt pause raised questions. Was it a moment of caution prompted by the admitting physician's inquiries about the diabetic status of the 93-year-old resident, or was it a calculated retreat, a prelude to more sinister deeds yet to unfold?

Pruning Shears with Charger

Martine, herself a nurse, noticed a disturbing shift in Kurt's demeanor following his mother's passing. Nocturnal restlessness gripped their once serene home, now tainted by Martine's bruised eyes and shattered kitchenware, evidence of Kurt's inexplicable outbursts of violence. As she grappled with the bewildering pattern of Kurt's job changes over the years, she couldn't shake the feeling that something dark was brewing beneath the surface.

Meanwhile, at work, Kurt seemed consumed by his duties, often found in the early hours with his head buried in his hands, lost in thought. Martine's unease deepened when she learned of the unsettling deaths occurring under Kurt's watch at the facility. Despite brushes with violence, including altercations with his own brother that led to a restraining order, patients continued to speak highly of Kurt's care.

Then, in the quiet of the night, Kurt's Internet search history revealed a chilling turn. He delved into the realms of liability, seeking answers about responsibility in the event of electrical mishaps with new appliances. This time, his actions were calculated, methodical. Yet, when confronted with evidence from his seized computer, Kurt deflected blame onto Martine, a desperate attempt to evade the encroaching shadows of his own malevolence.

Unbeknownst to her, she unwittingly played a role in this rather amateurish scheme. The next morning, Kurt instructed her to purchase an electric pruning shear with a charger, urgently. Later that same day, he ignited newspapers and hurled them at the newly acquired tool, setting the shed ablaze in a matter of moments. A neighbor's shout about smoke saved Kurt's wife and daughter, allowing them to narrowly escape the inferno that rendered their home uninhabitable, with damages totaling a staggering €267,121.

During the trial, the defendant claimed he intended to commit suicide, but his wife tearfully interjected during her testimony, suggesting that had anyone perished, it would have been herself and her daughter, as the arsonist callously observed from outside.

Ten days after the fire, Kurt injected an 82-year-old resident with a lethal dose of insulin. Deliberately delaying her transportation to the hospital by opting for non-emergency transport hours later instead of arranging for an ambulance, the woman narrowly escaped death. She courageously approached the stand during the trial, recounting her prolonged struggles with sleep and fear of being targeted again.

Despite offering apologies, the defendant appeared indifferent to her suffering, viewing himself as the victim. Confessing killing residents out of a warped sense of injustice over his mother and father-in-law's untimely deaths, contrasting their fate with the longevity of these elderly individuals.

Theatrical Deception

In the tense moments preceding his arrest, Kurt displayed an unexpected level of cooperation during his initial interrogation, adamantly denying any involvement in the insulin injections. However, as soon as the handcuffs clicked shut, a new narrative emerged, one involving the spectral voice of his deceased mother, purportedly guiding his every move. Suddenly claiming to possess a keen awareness of the residents' deaths occurring in his presence, attributing his actions to his mother's whispered commands.

Portraying himself as a mere pawn in a macabre game orchestrated by his late mother, Kurt described administering insulin doses as if playing a perilous round of Russian roulette, leaving fate to determine the dosage. With a flair for the dramatic, he would cast furtive glances towards the door, simulating apprehension at the mere thought of his mother's spectral presence. His portrayal was so convincing, it could have been lifted from a seasoned actor's playbook.

The nursing home's coordinator wove a tale of being forbidden sustenance by his phantom mother, a supposed consequence of his capture. Yet, without missing a beat, he resumed his normal eating habits, showing a remarkable ability to switch roles at will. Persistently demanding medical attention, he assumed the guise of a concerned patient in need of urgent care.

As night descended, he reached out to his father with tearful claims of a suicide attempt involving his belt. However, upon his father's arrival, his demeanor betrayed the falsity of his tale, revealing a calculated attempt to manipulate emotions. Martine, his wife, distanced herself from him after initiating divorce proceedings, choosing to sever all ties with the deceptive theatrics that had become Kurt's reality.

Chilling Verdict

Throughout the interrogation process, the nurse exhibits a stark refusal to cooperate on three crucial occasions. First, when a psychiatrist penetrates his hallucinations, noting that delusions don't suddenly arise posthumously but rather have roots in much earlier years. Second, Kurt balks at the idea of admitting himself to a psychiatric clinic during an emergency situation. Finally, when confronted with his training in 2004 for patients with diabetes, which should have endowed him with a comprehensive understanding of insulin dynamics.

In a succinct overview of the psychological and psychiatric evaluation, a chilling portrait emerges. The suspect displays a notable absence of emotion and remorse. Despite his attempts to portray a muddled psyche, the test results reveal a disturbingly normal level of concentration. However, his delayed responses to questions about hallucinations hint at deception. This man is characterized as a calculating murderer with psychopathic tendencies, including extreme deceitfulness, dominance, aggressive narcissism, manipulation, and persuasive charm. His actions are deemed fully accountable, rendering him a perpetual threat to society.

Following a unanimous guilty verdict from the entire jury, the seasoned judges of the Assize Court, alongside the jurors, decisively sentence Kurt Dobbelaere to life imprisonment. With the verdict sealed, there is no possibility of appeal after a verdict from the Assize Court.

21.

Tracing

Charles Cullen, United States, 1987

Curriculum Vitae

While the Netherlands only embraced professional registration for healthcare workers in 1996, North America had been pursuing this territory since 1970. However, delving into the annals of Charles Cullen's past you will discover a labyrinth of systemic shortcomings. It's a twisted story, made worse by the fragmented jurisdiction of the State Board of Nursing, which operates under a patchwork of state rules rather than a uniform national standard. This legal loophole provided Charles with an escape route; When it became too hot under his feet in New Jersey, he simply slipped across the border into Pennsylvania.

Beyond his nursing credentials lies a sixteen-year career path marred by tumultuous twists and turns, marked by a series of departures: dismissals from four branches, four voluntary departures, a forced dismissal and in an institution where he works through an employment agency, they no longer want to use his services.

A chilling testament to the dark underbelly of the healthcare profession, where the lines between healer and harbinger of harm blur into a sinister tapestry of malpractice and mayhem.

Misfortune

In the bleak dawn of a February morning in 1960, Charles entered the world prematurely, the youngest among eight siblings in a devout Catholic household. Their humble abode nestled in East Orange, a town along the bustling thoroughfare to the industrial area west of the Hudson River in the state of New Jersey. But life's cruel hand was swift to deal a blow; Charles barely had time to leave the incubator before his father succumbed to a grave illness.

Left to fend for themselves with only their mother as a provider, the family teetered on the edge of destitution. Their mother, a stoic figure, eked out a meager living scrubbing the homes of the more affluent while her children, led by the resilient older ones, shouldered the burden of caretaking. Yet, amidst this struggle, Charles, a sensitive soul, found solace in his mother's presence, yearning for her return every moment she was away.

As the years passed, Charles's inner turmoil grew. At the tender age of nine, he sought escape through a grim attempt at self-annihilation, swallowing chemicals in a desperate bid to flee his overwhelming reality.

His elementary and high school years relatively passing uneventfully. But tragedy, an ever-loyal companion, revisited the family when Charles was seventeen. Their matriarch, the beacon of strength in their stormy sea, perished in a tragic car accident, leaving the five remaining children adrift in a sea of uncertainty.

A Sailor's Struggle

At eighteen, Charles sought the allure of the sea and embarked on a journey with the United States Navy. Rising through the ranks, he earned the title of Third Class Technician, specializing in the intricate world of submarines, particularly those of the nuclear variety. But within the tight-knit quarters of the vessel, Charles found himself adrift amidst his peers. His lean frame made him an easy target for their jests, his only refuge being the sick bay where he offered a helping hand whenever his duties allowed.

On leave, Charles proudly donned his uniform, parading through the neighborhood with a façade of confidence. Yet beneath the polished exterior lurked a profound melancholy. Haunted by inner demons, he grappled with despair, a struggle that led him to a second suicide attempt with death and a reluctant admission to a psychiatric facility.

After serving six years in the navy, he is discharged for some obscure reason. Evil tongues claiming that, instead of being in the engine room, he was found in a doctor's coat, with a mouth patch and sterile gloves behind the control panel that can be used to fire atomic bombs.

At twenty-four, Charles found himself thrust back onto the shores of civilian life, liberated yet burdened by the weight of his past. With a newfound resolve, he redirected his focus toward a noble cause, the desire to lend a helping hand to those in need.

'The Shadow'

After his discharge from the Navy, Charles embarked on a new chapter in 1984, just eight kilometers north of his birthplace in the quaint town of Montclair, diving into the world of nursing, determined to carve out a career for himself. Yet, amidst the pursuit of his dreams, tragedy struck once more when his older brother tragically ended his life. Despite the heartache, Charles persevered and, three years later, proudly graduated with honors.

He married his girlfriend, a computer programmer and together, they settled into a comfortable home in Phillipsburg, nestled in the western reaches of New Jersey. Their family grew with the arrival of their first daughter, followed by another four years later.

As fatherhood beckoned, Charles secured a position at the most esteemed medical center in New Jersey, located in Livingston, a considerable ninety kilometers east of his home. His role in the burn unit seemed a promising start to his career. Colleagues and superiors alike admired his dedication, even as he predominantly worked night shifts, striving to please everyone with his eager demeanor. At the slightest sign of discomfort from a patient, Charles was ready with a syringe. Despite his outward charm, there lingered a subtle distance in Charles's interactions. After exhausting shifts, he retreated into solitude, his silence deafening. His demeanor at home grew increasingly brusque, his patience wearing thin with his wife and children, expecting his wife to carry heavy loads while pregnant and himself struggling with recurring bouts of depression.

As Charles navigated the complexities of his new career, a chilling incident cast a shadow over the burn unit. The inexplicable death of a seventy-two-year-old man under his watch raised eyebrows, yet was dismissed as an unfortunate occurrence, a mere footnote in the chaos of a hospital's daily operations.

Off-duty, Charles sought solace in the numbing embrace of alcohol, drowning his troubles in cans of beer. His daytime sleep was restless, disrupting the daily routine of his household, much to the dismay of his wife, struggling to maintain order amidst the chaos of motherhood.

After two years, Charles bids farewell to his post and transitions into part-time work at the hospital through a staffing agency, assuming the role of a versatile 'float' employee, available to assist in various departments. His shifts stretch from dusk till dawn, a nocturnal existence that mirrors his inner turmoil.

His penchant for alcohol begins to blur the lines between his professional and personal life, leading to brushes with the law for reckless driving. Even at home, his wife's criticisms are met with violence, revealing cracks in his once-veneered facade of normalcy.

As he traverses the hospital corridors during his nightly shifts, Charles becomes a spectral figure, earning the nickname 'the Shadow' among his peers. His solitary figure, shrouded in the darkness, conceals a tumultuous inner world haunted by financial strain and existential despair.

In moments of solitude, he grapples with the weight of his responsibilities, contemplating drastic measures to escape his mounting burdens. Yet, even as he battles his inner demons, he remains dedicated to his duties, faithfully tending to the needs of patients while his own life unravels.

Sitting for hours, lost in melancholy. With two children and hefty mortgage payments, struggling to make ends meet despite his efforts. Consumed by despair, he ingests a handful of pills, leading to a hospitalization where his stomach is pumped. A week later, he resumes his rounds among hospital beds.

Another mysterious death occurs, establishing insulin in the intravenous fluid of a patient who isn't diabetic, followed by an investigation ensues. As whispers of suspicion circulate, Charles's tenure as a temporary staff member abruptly comes to an end, shrouded in secrecy and suspicion. The hospital's decision to distance itself from him speaks volumes, leaving behind unanswered questions and a lingering sense of unease in the wake of 'The Shadow's' enigmatic presence. The hospital keeps the assumption under wraps, never disclosing it to the public.

Children's Books

In a nation grappling with a dire shortage of nurses in the tumultuous year of 1992, hospitals clamored for every available pair of hands. It was amidst this chaotic backdrop that Charles found himself sought after, transitioning seamlessly from one institution to another. Barely a month had passed since his departure from his initial workplace when he landed a position at a local hospital in Phillipsburg, his hometown.

Nestled within the walls of this modern regional hospital, with its array of 200 beds, Charles embarked on a journey fraught with both professional duties and personal turmoil. Tasked with the demanding responsibilities of the intensive care and cardiac units, he also grappled with the looming shadow of his brother's diagnosis, diagnosed with a brain tumor, a grim reminder of life's fragility.

Yet, beyond the sterile confines of hospital corridors, Charles's life unfurled in a tapestry of darkness. The fabric of his marriage, once woven with hope and promise, began to unravel amidst a tempest of domestic violence and emotional turmoil. His wife, driven to desperation, sought refuge in the arms of the law, painting a harrowing portrait of her husband's descent into madness.

With chilling detail, she recounted tales of horror, her husband's bizarre and violent behavior, including gouging out the eye of their cat, Mickey, and mutilating the ear of their dog, Shirley, before callously disposing of the injured animal in the trash. During a visit from a friend and her husband, Charles allegedly spiked their drinks with gasoline. Furthermore, he set fire to his daughter's reading books in the backyard and reportedly inquired about funeral rates from undertakers. But amidst the litany of accusations, one incident pierced through the veil of disbelief, the abandonment of their daughters in the care of a stranger for days on end, as their mother lay hospitalized, vulnerable and alone.

For Charles, the path forward was bleak, with no choice but to flee the family home and seek refuge in a nearby rental. Custody of his children fell to his wife, a decision influenced by Charles's troubled past marred by abuse, depression, and multiple suicide attempts. His visits with his daughters were strictly supervised, overshadowed by the looming threat of legal action for his failure to provide financial support.

In a spiral of despair, Charles found himself once again on the precipice of self-destruction, his fourth suicide attempt landing him in the confines of a regional medical center's behavioral disorders unit.

Still, even within the confines of these grim walls, Charles's woes continued to mount. Desperate to escape the suffocating grip of financial ruin, he toiled relentlessly, adding an extra burden of 12 to 36 hours of work each week to his already taxing night shift duties. His choice of patients, those teetering on the brink of death, raising eyebrows among his colleagues, who regarded him with a mixture of suspicion and unease.

As Charles shuffled through the dimly lit corridors of the hospital, his presence evoked a sense of foreboding among those who crossed his path. Muttering softly to himself, he appeared lost in a private torment, a haunting figure that left his colleagues on edge. Yet, amidst the darkness that surrounded him, two elderly women met their untimely demise under circumstances that left lingering questions in their wake.

Stalking

Love, that fickle and treacherous emotion, ensnares Charles once again, weaving a tangled web of desire and obsession. His heart swells with affection for a colleague, but her icy indifference ignites a dangerous spark within him. Ignoring her pleas for space, he descends into a relentless pursuit, a twisted dance that culminates in a chilling intrusion into her sanctuary as she slumbers, his desperate attempts to win her favor marked by the theft of trinkets and tokens of her existence.

But fate is not blind to his deeds, and soon the consequences come knocking at his door. Despite the gravity of his transgressions, Charles manages to skirt the jaws of justice, receiving a mere slap on the wrist in the form of a suspended sentence, a hefty fine, and a restraining order.

In addition, the sting of rejection fuels his descent into darkness, plunging him deeper into the abyss of despair. In a desperate bid to escape his torment, he embraces the finality of oblivion, sealing himself in his garage with the engine roaring, a macabre ode to the agony that consumes him.

Rushed to the hospital where he once walked the halls as a healer, his colleagues now rally around him as he is shuttled between successive psychiatric institutions, each a pitstop on his journey through the labyrinth of his tortured mind.

Forced into outpatient therapy by his employer under threat of termination, Charles's return to work is met with unexpected complications. The family of a patient whose death occurred under suspicious circumstances initiates legal proceedings against him. Allegations of injecting a dying woman with a mysterious substance, draining the color from her face as life slipped away, cast a dark shadow over his once-promising career.

As scrutiny intensifies, Charles is engulfed in a whirlwind of accusations and investigations. Although the attempted murder charge ultimately fails due to lack of evidence, the hospital's failure to report the incident to the New Jersey State Nursing Board adds fuel to the growing fire. Charles feels the walls around him closing in and takes matters into his own hands. He resigns after a tumultuous tenure of more than a year and a half.

Fueled by Impulse

In a whirlwind of change, Charles swiftly returns to the workforce within a mere four months, this time finding himself in the embrace of the third institution, situated 25 miles southeast. Nestled amidst the serene landscapes of Flemington, a picturesque town along the banks of the Delaware River Valley, this quaint hospital boasting 176 beds also houses a prestigious oncology center. Once again, Charles is tasked with the responsibilities of the intensive care unit, details are carefully checked when applying. According to the Board of Nursing in New Jersey, his reputation cannot be faulted. Previous hospital admissions or psychiatric treatment remain undiscussed.

For eight months, Charles devotes himself diligently to his duties in Flemington, until a tempest of passion ignites within him, leading to a clandestine affair with a married colleague. Despite his steadfast adherence to antidepressant medication, the initial eighteen months at this hospital pass without incident, with Charles even earning commendation for his dedication. Yet, when the flames of romance are extinguished abruptly by his girlfriend's departure after nearly two years, a sinister pattern emerges. Within the span of six short months, five unsuspecting patients meet their untimely death. Fueled by a surge of impulsive decision-making, Charles submits his resignation in haste, only to reconsider his actions in the aftermath. However, the hospital administration remains steadfast in their decision, citing his entanglement with a married colleague as the primary catalyst for his dismissal.

Animal Welfare

No need to panic, for there are plenty of healthcare facilities to choose from. Charles ventures 50 kilometers southeast, and within two weeks, he secures a position at the fourth institution, a hospital boasting over

500 beds, located in Morristown. Here, he settles into a gloomy-looking abode, seeking solace in the companionship of a ferret and a dog. However, in his neglect, he leaves them chained outside in freezing temperatures. Concerned neighbors alert the animal welfare authorities, resulting in the removal of the animals and a hefty fine for the nurse.

Frustrated and weighed down by the heavy burden of alimony obligations, Charles finds himself teetering on the edge once more. The stress of his predicament triggers a distressing pattern of misconduct within the hospital walls. He tampers with vital medical equipment, disrupts medication regimens, and defiantly disregards the orders of attending physicians. As a consequence of his actions, his employment contract is abruptly terminated after a mere ten months.

While no lives are lost under his care at this institution, a deafening silence ensues regarding his professional failings. The New Jersey State Nursing Board remains oblivious to his lapses in competence, allowing Charles to slip through the cracks of accountability.

With the dust of professional upheaval settling around him, Charles, now 37 years old, finds himself adrift in a sea of uncertainty, navigating the turbulent waters of unemployment for two long months.

Questions

Amidst the lull of unemployment, Charles takes a strategic step, obtaining his registration to practice in the neighboring state of Pennsylvania, where his slate remains untainted by the scandalous professional behavior of his past.

With newfound credentials in hand, he embarks on a journey westward, crossing state lines to rendezvous with his fifth institution, a blend of nursing home and rehabilitation center nestled in Allentown, a mere 150 kilometers from his former haunt. The facility, aching for skilled hands, eagerly slots him into the nocturnal rhythms of the respiratory care unit.

Yet, as swiftly as the night descends, the façade of competence begins to crumble. Mere months into his tenure, whispers of suspicion permeate the corridors as Charles is spotted slipping into a patient's chamber with an incongruous pair of loaded syringes. The aftermath reveals a scene of chaos: a distressed patient, a fractured limb, and bed linens tangled in disarray.

Caught in the act of tampering with another patient's respirator, Charles skillfully maneuvers his way out of trouble with a clever excuse. However, the vanishing act of vials from the medication vault raises eyebrows among his vigilant peers.

Questions linger like whispers in the night: why would a seasoned ICU veteran like Charles accept a position in a nursing home, a perceived demotion in the hierarchy of healthcare? And why Allentown, a locale far removed from his domicile, when closer hospitals beckon with the allure of higher wages?

In the wake of an unexpected demise, an 83-year-old man lies motionless, his body tainted by an overdose of insulin. Initially, blame falls on another nurse for administering a misguided injection. However, she points the finger at Charles as the perpetrator, filing a lawsuit against the hospital for false allegations.

Eight months later, Charles finds himself ousted from his position. The institution, in an attempt to cleanse its tarnished reputation, dutifully reports to the Department of Health the termination of their former employee, Mr. Cullen, citing improper medication administration as the cause. However, the governing body overseeing all nursing homes in Pennsylvania lacks the jurisdiction to hold individual nurses accountable. Thus, neither the police nor the State Board of Nursing of Pennsylvania are alerted to Charles's transgressions.

For Charles Cullen, this is just another chapter in a tumultuous journey. Within a mere eleven years since his graduation, he has traversed through the halls of five different institutions, enduring termination of employment twice under shrouded circumstances and facing dismissal once. His existence is marred by the specter of pain, with five suicide attempts, along with enduring five psychiatric admissions. Amidst the turmoil, he has faced three charges, culminating in a single conviction.

But the tally doesn't conclude with five institutions; Charles Cullen's indelible mark spans across ten, leaving behind a trail of uncertainty, suspicion, and tragedy.

Doubt

In the blink of an eye, the nurse found himself without a job. With pockets pinched, he swiftly signed up with a temp agency in Easton, a small town a good twenty miles down the road in Pennsylvania. Desperate for cash flow, he didn't hesitate to juggle roles in not one but two facilities through this agency. His first stop, the sixth institution on his list, was a hospital right in Easton, where he plunged into full-time night shifts in the intensive care unit.

It didn't take long for the clock to run out on an 87-year-old man, a mere month into his stint. His daughter, sitting vigil, watched a pallid nurse administer what seemed like an ominous injection just moments before her father's final breath. After an autopsy, the district pathologist was left with persistent doubts.

Supervisors and doctors found solace in a simple narrative: an unnamed nurse must have made a tragic mistake, overdosing the patient. It's the age-old tale of least resistance, powered by the haunting specter of litigation, a common occurrence in a land where wrongful accusations often lead to hefty settlements.

When journalists sought clarity from the hospital about any inquiries into nurse Charles Cullen's involvement, the response was shrouded in silence. But hushed whispers among former colleagues painted a different picture, suggesting that he was indeed the one who wielded the syringe, administering the fateful dose of heart stimulant.

Feeling the noose tightening, Charles made his hasty exit after a mere four months. And amidst the chaos, he found solace in the fleeting moments spent by his brother's side, a soul already slipping into the reality of his last phase.

Fire

In a whirlwind of activity, Charles swiftly transitioned from his stint at the sixth institution to a part-time position at his seventh stop, a hospital nestled in the heart of Allentown. Here, once again, he found himself tending to the wounded souls of the burn unit. Allentown held no secrets for him, for it was only two short months ago that he bid adieu to the nursing home and detox clinic nearby. With his departure from the sixth institution, he now plunged headlong into the full-time rhythm of this new workplace.

Authorities, in their customary manner, went through the motions of vetting Charles's references from the fifth institution, the nearby nursing home and detox clinic. However, the unsavory details of his dismissal remained shrouded in silence. Consequently, the seventh institution remained blissfully ignorant of the peril they invited by welcoming this nurse into their ranks. It didn't take long for the first ripple of concern to emerge. Despite a promising outlook for a 22-year-old patient, she was abruptly torn from the fabric of life. A natural death certificate was the unfortunate conclusion.

Now, for the sixth time, Charles attempted suicide by setting fire in his bathtub, hoping the smoke would suffocate him. Local law enforcement, prompted by the watchful eyes of vigilant neighbors, discovered him in a disoriented state. Charles spun a tale of seeking solace from the chilling grasp of the night, a narrative that failed to quell the officers' growing unease. Their subsequent inspection of his dwelling revealed a stark reality, a barren abode stripped of life's comforts, save for a meager assortment of furnishings and children's drawings adorning the walls. The revelation that this trembling soul was registered as a certified nurse, tasked with tending to the delicate souls of a burn unit, left them reeling.

Transported to a crisis center against his better judgment, Charles soon charted his own course, only to find himself back within the confines of its walls shortly thereafter. In a cruel twist of fate, barely a month elapsed before he resumed his nocturnal duties within the burn unit's hallowed halls. It was there that a 73-year-old woman teetered on the precipice of death, her fate sealed a mere five days later.

Sixteen tumultuous months later, discounting the turbulent days spent within the confines of the crisis center, Charles bid a somber farewell to the burn unit, his tenure marked by whispers of tragedy and unanswered questions, never to return.

Pandemic of Suspicion

For the following two months, Charles devoted himself to the care of his ailing brother, a solemn duty that culminated in his passing in June 2000. With meticulous care, Charles orchestrated the funeral arrangements, a final act of love for his departed kin. Yet, even amidst the shroud of grief, the call to return to the fray beckoned him.

The perpetual shortage of healthcare personnel persisted unabated, casting its shadow over countless institutions. Thus, when Charles found himself in the employ of the eighth institution, another cog in the vast machinery of healthcare, he did so via an intermediary, a staffing agency that, in the customary manner, reached out to his former workplaces for references. Yet, as tradition dictated, the seventh and fifth institutions provided little more than a snapshot of his tenure, their records silent on anything beyond the start and end dates of his employment. At the age of forty, Charles embarked on a new chapter within the halls of the eighth institution, a sprawling healthcare center nestled in Bethlehem, boasting a workforce of five thousand souls. Situated halfway between Allentown and Easton, this establishment welcomed Charles into its fold, assigning him to the nine-bed heart monitoring unit, a domain where life teetered on the edge of fragility. Here, amidst the beeping monitors and hushed whispers of uncertainty, Charles found solace in the camaraderie of his colleagues, occasionally venturing beyond the confines of the hospital to partake in the shared experience of cultural outings, perhaps seeking respite from the weight of his somber duties. A gesture of kindness towards a colleague who had recently given birth, presenting her with a gift of a baby blanket, spoke volumes of Charles's ostensibly caring nature.

Yet, the specter of suspicion refused to be banished from his doorstep. Eight months into his tenure at the eighth institution, another life was snuffed out under murky circumstances. Meanwhile, a looming threat awaited him at home, a lawsuit stemming from the wrongful accusation levied against a colleague during his time at the fifth institution.

In due time, the wheels of justice fail to connect Charles to the passing of the 83-year-old patient, whose bloodstream swam with an alarming excess of insulin. Seeking clarity, an investigator reaches out to Charles's current workplace, the eighth institution. But Human Resources, veiling Charles's status as a contractual worker through a staffing agency, denies any trace of his presence on their official roster.

Across eleven months, commencing in June 2001, a perplexing saga unfolds as five patients, unexpectedly expired, while reclined in their hospital beds. One succumbs after a single resuscitation attempt, while another endures four, before succumbing to the ultimate fate. Charles's conspicuous attendance at these somber scenes does not evade scrutiny. Swift to console grieving families, he displays a peculiar eagerness in the aftermath of each tragedy. Moreover, amidst the chaos, discarded ampoules of an unauthorized heart stimulant surface in the sharps bin, a medication undocumented in any patient's regimen. Amongst colleagues, murmurs escalate as the incidence of resuscitations and fatalities skyrockets, doubling from the usual count of ten to eleven per month.

Summoned to account for his actions, Charles retreats into denial, steadfastly withholding any admission of involvement. However, one astute nurse, meticulously chronicling the chain of deaths, reveals that Charles was on duty during a staggering 60 percent of these suspicious fatalities.

Just a month later, as yet another patient meets a dubious end, the meticulous nurse, burdened by her findings, reaches a tipping point. She takes her concerns to the Pennsylvania State Nursing Board, igniting an internal inquiry into the administration of questionable medications.

Never the less, come June 2002, instead of facing termination, Charles is permitted to 'resign' from his role at the eighth institution. Though the institution discloses Charles's suspected misconduct to the Board, he vehemently rebuffs all allegations. And with tangible evidence eluding the investigation, the hospital evades any punitive measures.

In the wake of his departure from the eighth institution, lingering whispers persist, nourished by speculation surrounding the abrupt cessation of the resuscitation and fatality epidemic that seemingly coincided with Charles's exit.

Coincidence

In a twist of fate, Charles, now 42, swiftly finds himself back in the fold within a month, securing a position at the ninth establishment, a Catholic hospital once more in Allentown, a place he had frequented twice before. His reentry into the medical realm commences with a mandated eight-week orientation program.

Just a scant sixteen days into the training, while on duty in a hospital ward, Charles encounters the colleague who had previously leveled false accusations against him. Startled by her unexpected presence, she promptly alerts the administration to Charles's alleged involvement in a prior medication mishap under ongoing investigation.

He is swiftly asked to leave, officially reprimanded for his purportedly poor interpersonal skills and deemed guilty of unprofessional behavior.

Curiously, the hospital administration opts not to notify the Pennsylvania State Nursing Board of this incident. Nevertheless, an article surfaces in the local newspaper, shedding light on the ongoing investigation and igniting a spark of recognition among Charles's former colleagues.

As the pressure mounts and scrutiny intensifies, the district pathologist, harboring lingering doubts about the circumstances surrounding a previous death at the sixth institution, joins the unfolding drama. Despite an investigative committee's thorough questioning of numerous concerned nurses, Charles miraculously evades direct interrogation, for reasons unknown, Charles remains exempt from their scrutiny.

Total Loss

Within a mere eight weeks, the seasoned nurse finds himself back in the whirlwind of hospital life, this time within the bustling confines of the tenth institution, a sprawling university hospital nestled in Somerville, a distant 96 kilometers to the east in New Jersey.

Though Charles may have vanished from sight, the echoes of his past deeds still reverberate in the corridors of Pennsylvania's medical facilities. The administration of the eighth institution in Bethlehem wastes no time in officially reporting him to the Board, citing suspicions of pilfering medications for reasons yet undisclosed. Prompted by this alarming report, the Board swiftly mobilizes law enforcement to initiate a thorough investigation.

However, as fate would have it, Charles's current employer remains oblivious. Unaware of the storm brewing, the hospital continues its operations, blissfully ignorant of the looming threat. Meanwhile, Charles, ever the master of deception, conveniently omits any mention of his employment at the ninth institution from his application form, ensuring his past remains shrouded in secrecy.

On a fateful September day in 2002, Charles steps foot into the hallowed halls of the intensive care unit, ready to resume his duties. However, the modern trappings of this hospital present an unexpected hurdle for the seasoned nurse. The introduction of a sophisticated computerized medication dispensing system poses a challenge, casting a shadow of doubt on Charles's meticulously crafted schemes. He realizes, with a sinking heart, that the very drugs he once wielded with impunity can now be traced with alarming ease.

As the days pass, Charles's once meticulous facade begins to crack. Within a mere 156 days of his employment, tragedy strikes. In the dead of night, mere moments following his 43rd birthday, two patients draw their last breaths.

The cunning nurse has devised a clever method to circumvent the computerized system. Under the cover of darkness, he enters the medication room, punches in his login code and the purported prescription on the computer screen. As the medication drawer slides open, he swiftly pockets the ampule into his uniform, canceling the request before closing the drawer, erasing any trace of the missing medication.

But even the most carefully laid plans are not immune to scrutiny. Charles's reckless actions draw attention, casting a spotlight on his clandestine activities. Within a mere thirteen weeks, three more patients succumb to the shadows, their deaths shrouded in mystery, their fates entwined with that of the enigmatic nurse.

Almost Caught

Yet, Charles has since moved in with a woman who has two children of her own, an unsettling pattern of inexplicable deaths continues. Just nine days removed from the last somber occasion, the sterile halls of the hospital witness the harrowing struggle of a 21-year-old patient, his young heart faltering thrice in rapid succession before the vigilant efforts of medical staff manage to reclaim him from the brink each time. Between each tumultuous resuscitation, the nurse, with a disturbing casualness, regales the stricken parents with vivid, morbid details of their son's desperate dance with mortality. The parents, shaken to their core by these grim narratives, hastily bid the nurse farewell, their hearts heavy with the weight of impending loss. It is in the hushed moments of the fourth resuscitation attempt, as the mother's tearful plea to let her son die peacefully, acknowledging the irreversible damage to his brain function.

The joint investigation by the Board and the police has now reached Charles' current employer, but the tenth institution remains silent as long as possible. They would have been better off not doing that, because within seven days of the joint research starting in this tenth institution, two patients showed symptoms of an insulin overdose. And another twelve days later, a forty-year-old man suddenly needs cardiac massage again, during which a high dose of cardiac stimulant is found in his blood. Two bottles of the same medicine are missing.

After more than a week, a postoperative patient, a priest, dies unexpectedly, who, like the previous victim, was not under Charles' responsibility. Once again, a high concentration of the heart stimulant is found in the priest's blood. The relatives refuse an autopsy, but the hospital management becomes concerned. Ultimately, it will be the unexpected death of this priest that will throw the whole thing off for Charles.

Over a week later, a post-surgical patient, a priest, breathes his last breath, falling victim to circumstances beyond Charles's direct care, similar to the previous casualty.

Once again, an elevated concentration of the heart stimulant is detected in the priest's bloodstream. Despite the family's refusal for an autopsy, the hospital administration grows increasingly concerned. Ultimately, it is the unexpected parting of this priest that sets the entire investigation into motion, unraveling the tangled web spun by Charles.

Brutal

In the sultry heat of midsummer, the tenth institution, grappling with yet more inexplicable deaths, brazenly hires a private investigator to unravel the enigma surrounding the sudden surge in resuscitations. As the investigator meticulously pores over digital records, each resuscitation or demise inexorably linked to Charles Cullen's canceled medication orders, the hospital remains obstinate in retaining him. Meanwhile, the resuscitation team is summoned six more times, their efforts yielding a mixed bag of outcomes.

Despite the ominous cloud cast by the untimely passing of the priest, three months go by before the hospital begrudgingly notifies the district attorney of their suspicions of nefarious involvement in matters of mortality. With the arrival of two detectives on the ward, Charles finds himself unceremoniously fired, his departure ostensibly veiled by alleged falsifications on his employment application.

Undeterred by the glaring scrutiny of the media and the impending specter of law enforcement, Charles audaciously ventures into the halls of yet another institution, a mere eleven miles away. Within its familiar walls, he seeks solace, once finding refuge following his third suicide.

As December dawns, local and international media outlets buzz with speculation and dread. For the intrepid private detective and determined law enforcement, the truth becomes apparent with chilling swiftness: Charles, the nurse shrouded in darkness, stands as the focal point of their investigation, his presence looming large over the corridors of healing.

Puzzle Pieces

On December 12, 2003, as the summer sun shone brightly, Charles was taken into custody upon leaving a restaurant where he had dined on unlimited spare ribs with his girlfriend. Upon his arrival at the police station, he hesitated before beginning to confess in fits and starts to the deaths of numerous patients that weighed heavily on his conscience. As described in Clifford and Martin's gripping book *Death Angel* (2005), suspects of grave crimes often exhibit repetitive speech patterns, faltering and restarting, speaking in fragments, stuttering, gasping for breath, only to resume their narrative again.

After his initial outpouring, Charles fell silent for an extended period. Early on in the extensive investigation, it emerged that the suspect had previously come under suspicion on several occasions.

Ultimately, Charles became cooperative in assembling the puzzle pieces. He compiled a list of key points to expedite the capture of future perpetrators, in exchange for a waiver from the death penalty. Which might not demonstrate a nuanced comprehension, but a true cynic might remark on this bargain that it's a curious step for someone who attempted to end his own life six times. And further, how peculiar it is that someone adept at extinguishing others' lives failed to extinguish his own?

To a psychiatrist, Charles would later confide that most of the murders were impulsive acts. In other instances, he meticulously planned the killings, consciously selecting victims whose deaths would attract the least attention. Instead of directing his desire for death towards himself, he directed it towards others. Additionally, he claimed to have always lived with the fear of being discovered. However, that fear diminished as he convinced himself that he was relieving the suffering of the patient.

According to Michael Welner, a New York-based professor of psychiatry and an expert on serial killers, killing out of compassion is a rationalization that perpetrators use to convince themselves they've done something good. Charles wasn't entirely devoid of conscience, as he occasionally grappled with intense guilt, although never enough to halt his actions. Apparently, the pride of remaining undetected for so long outweighed any guilt he experienced.

In 2006, Charles Cullen was convicted of thirteen murders, two attempted murders, and forty suspected murders. Using, as far as known, eight different types of medication, with a heart stimulant being the most common choice.

As the emotionally charged trial came to a close, he refused to utter a final word. From the balcony, bereaved family members unleashed their anger towards the defendant's bench, but Charles remained silent.

As the verdict of eleven life sentences was pronounced, the 46-year-old man, wearing a bulletproof vest beneath his sweater for protection against the enraged public, kept his eyes shut.

While this book has primarily focused on cases involving nursing and healthcare personnel, as well as a respiratory therapist, committing crimes against their patients, it is important to note that serial killers may also lurk among medical physicians. The concluding chapters of this book delve into doctors, beginning with the unsettling tale of an American physician who ventured as a serial killer in as far as Africa, operating in a modest mission hospital.

22.

Crossing borders

Michael Swango, United States, 1970

Goodbye

In the hazy heat of May 1995, tragedy struck the humble abode of a woman in Mnene, Zimbabwe. It was no ordinary mishap that befell her, but a scalding accident involving a pot of steaming maize porridge. The searing burns she suffered became her ticket to the Lutheran mission hospital, nestled in the heart of what was once known as Rhodesia, a territory steeped in colonial history.

Despite the skilled hands of the medical staff, fate played a cruel hand. Just as hope began to flicker within the sterile walls of the hospital, the woman was found lifeless in her bed, a sudden and perplexing demise that left the medical director puzzled, but knowing better than anyone that death is never far away in his hospital. He files away her patient records and forgets about the incident.

Meanwhile, amidst the lingering scent of antiseptic and fear, another patient found himself at the mercy of a peculiar doctor named Mike, an white American whose methods raised eyebrows among the locals. In the aftermath of an appendectomy, the man awoke to the chilling sight of Doctor Mike, wielding a syringe with practiced ease. What followed was a series of events shrouded in suspicion and deceit, leaving the patient paralyzed and his future hanging by a thread. Hearing the doctor say

'Goodbye' before quickly leaving the ward. But Doctor Mike denies the injection vehemently and claims the patient was delirious. The consequences for the patient, whose condition significantly worsened after the injection, are considerable. After a nasty infection, his lower leg has to be amputated, depriving him of his ability to work his piece of land for much longer.

A month later, in the sweltering heat of a Zimbabwean afternoon, the hospital corridors buzzed with activity, yet within the confines of one room, a tragedy unfolded that would send shockwaves through the community. A traffic accident victim lay in his bed, surrounded by his bustling family. As the aroma of pancakes filled the air, a scene of normalcy clashed with the undercurrent of unease. The arrival of Doctor Mike, a figure of authority tinged with suspicion, only added to the tension. With a wave of his hand, he dismissed the family, leaving them to wonder at the screams that pierced through the thin veil of the bed curtain.

It was a scene straight out of a nightmare as the patient's wife hesitated, her fear palpable, waiting for the doctor's departure, disregarding her inquiries, before daring to approach her husband. Yet, even as she reached his side, his mutterings of impending doom echoed in her ears, a grim premonition of the tragedy to come. Murmuring that his end draws near after a prick. Hours later, the man succumbs to death's embrace.

As the family mourned their loss, their cries of anguish reverberating through their humble home, questions lingered unanswered. How could a man, seemingly on the road to recovery, meet such a sudden loss of life? And why did the doctor's presence seem to cast a shadow over their grief-stricken hearts? Complaints falling on def ears, cause no injection was administered. A family navigating life without its breadwinner. As they bid farewell to the deceased in their corrugated iron abode the following day, the women collapse onto the ground in loud wails.

Amidst the darkness, another tale of despair unfolded. A farmer's wife, her husband's amputated foot a stark reminder of their shattered dreams, found herself alone in the silent hours of the night. Living 48 hours' walk away from the hospital, allowing to stay overnight. Just before extinguishing the light, they discuss their future plans. In the dead of night, the woman catches sight of a white doctor approaching her husband's bed. Assuming the doctor is merely conducting a routine check, she drifts back to sleep, only to be roused when a nurse taps her shoulder. Does she even realize her husband has passed away?

And then there was a pregnant woman, her anticipation overshadowed by dread as a blonde doctor approached with an air of secrecy. Without explanation, he administered an injection, plunging her into a world of agony and fear as flames seemed to engulf her, leaving her writhing in intense pain. Desperately, the woman begs for wet cloths to cool herself down. Shortly after the child is born, the nurse confronts the blonde doctor about what he injected. He denies any wrongdoing, and both mother and child eventually recover.

As days passed, the hospital's halls echoed with whispers of tragedy. A patient, weakened by an injection, crawled out of the hospital only to meet his end soon after, leaving behind a shattered family of five children. At his funeral, his niece, a hospital staff member fell victim to a mysterious illness, her symptoms worsening despite seeking help from the very doctor implicated in the previous tragedies. Sixty minutes later, she breathes her last.

Then, just a week later, a woman arrived, her life hanging by a thread bleeding profusely. After surgery under anesthesia removing miscarriage remnants, she fails to survive the night, leaving behind a hospital staff reeling from the series of inexplicable deaths.

Meanwhile the Swedish-born medical director is getting nervous. So many unexpected deaths, each involving his American colleague, haven't escaped his notice. He himself brought the man over from the States nine months ago, considering him a fine fellow with whom he had formed a friendship. Mike being charming company during dinners at the medical director's home, a captivating individual who held everyone enthralled.

In hindsight, it would have been wiser for the medical director to scrutinize the newcomer's credentials and references before unleashing him upon patients or to interrogate the American more thoroughly. Thanks to the book *Blind Eye, a Terrifying Story of a Doctor Who Got Away with Murder*, by James B. Stewart, we can uncover the identity of this enigmatic figure.

Treasured Son

In the heart of Tacoma, on a military base nestled amid the pine-scented forests of Washington, DC, the Swango family welcomed their second son into the world in the year 1954. They christened him Michael. Born into a world of military order and familial complexity, Michael's early years unfolded amidst the shifting sands of his parents' second marriages.

From the moment he drew his first breath, Michael's mother saw in him the promise of greatness, showering him with adoration throughout his formative years. But beneath the surface of this maternal affection lay the seeds of a future darker than anyone could have imagined. According to renowned forensic psychologist Dr. Jeffrey Smalldon, Michael's upbringing, coupled with his mother's excessive praise, would sow the seeds of a narcissism so profound it would lead him down a path of darkness. Father's militaristic upbringing, a stern military man serving in the tumult of Vietnam. Who's sporadic appearances were marked by strict discipline, he and his brother being forced to march and salute at his command. The growing boy losing sight of his normal self-image due to mothers excessively praising, developing an extreme form of narcissism. Moreover, the distant atmosphere at home and cold relationship between the parents. Never as a family together at the table. Both parents chain smokers.

When Michael is thirteen years old, after several moves across America, the family settles in Quincy, a town in the eastern state of Illinois. The mother works as an administrative assistant at a general practitioner's office, helping the children with their homework and reading bedtime stories. But all her attention cannot compensate for the lack of paternal love.

Michael's father skipping his leave and living with a Vietnamese woman in Southeast Asia. But when he does appear in Quincy, the strict regime is continued. The rare occasions when visitors come, both brothers stand guard, saluting at the door until they are excused. And not only mother suffers from father's loose hands, but the boys also bear the brunt. Father drinks, just like Michael's mother's first husband. When Michael excels in his high school diploma and his bachelor's degree with flying colors and signs up for the navy at the age of 21, his mother kicks her husband out, though never officially divorcing him.

Oddball

In the annals of college lore, Michael stood out as a peculiar figure from the outset. A romantic misfortune led to an eccentric transformation and by an unwavering fascination with all things military. Eschewing conventional attire, he draped himself in military garb and even repainted his once ordinary Ford Fairlane in shades of army green. But it was his macabre hobby that truly set him apart, collecting clippings of gravely wounded soldiers, a grim pastime that left his peers bewildered and distanced.

Despite his social estrangement, Michael remained undeterred in his ambitions. Discharged from the Marines under ambiguous circumstances, he redirected his focus toward a lofty goal: becoming a doctor. Enrolling in medical school back in Quincy, his hometown, Michael embellishing his application receiving two medals for heroism in the Marines.

Remarkably, Michael excelled academically, despite the demands of his studies and his concurrent employment as a nursing assistant in a local hospital, obtaining a certification as an ambulance nurse. His proficiency in the medical field was as impressive as it was unexpected, earning him certifications and accolades that belied his peculiarities.

Yet, amidst the academic rigor, Michael's interests took a dark turn. In a dissertation that foreshadowed his own sinister deeds, he delved into the chilling assassination of Bulgarian writer Georgi Markov, who had been assassinated in exile in London. Given Michael's later actions, it's worth delving into this case further.

As Georgi Markov walked across the English Waterloo Bridge over the Thames, he felt a sharp pain in his thigh. A man who had bumped into him retrieved his umbrella. Markov became violently ill and died a few days later. During his autopsy, a microscopic capsule containing ricin, an extremely toxic substance that causes blood to clot throughout the body, was found in his thigh. It's notable that Michael's interest in this case predates his own nefarious deeds by seven years.

At 24, Michael emerged from university halls with flying colors, adorned with the prestigious American Chemical Society Award as a testament to his academic prowess. His journey took him southward, to a university nestled in the heart of Illinois, where his aspirations collided with the reality of patient care. To his peers' bewilderment, Michael seemed untouched by the human aspect of medicine, his interactions with patients devoid of warmth or empathy. His swift intake assessments left his fellow students questioning the depth of his engagement, suspecting he merely scribbled notes without genuine concern.

Amongst whispers of concern, a group of five students grappled with the notion of reporting Michael's peculiar behavior. Yet, plagued by the fear of unjustly besmirching his reputation, they hesitated, allowing his enigmatic presence to linger unchallenged. Meanwhile, Michael's eccentricities persisted, his penchant for impromptu push-ups and attending lectures dressed in military attire, complete with combat boots, a sight that amused his classmates, mostly draft dodgers who had refused to fight in Vietnam. Plus, Michael displayed a particular fascination with toxicology, further adding to the mystery surrounding his intentions.

Fabrications

In the hallowed halls of medical academia, where students tread the delicate line between life and death, Michael's presence stirred whispers of unease. Assigned the solemn task of dissecting cadavers, his methods veered into the realm of the macabre. Under the cloak of darkness, he wielded a chainsaw with a chilling fervor, defying convention and sending shivers down the spines of his peers.

But Michael's peculiarities extended far beyond the confines of the anatomy lab. A chilling pattern emerged, patients who garnered his fleeting attention often met grim fates shortly thereafter, earning him the moniker 'Double-O-Swango', a nod to James Bond's infamous codename '007'.

Yet, it wasn't just his morbid fascination that set him apart. Driven by an insatiable energy, he defied the need for sleep, immersing himself in his studies with a fervor unmatched by his peers. And while rules forbade outside employment, Michael clandestinely moonlighted as an ambulance nurse, regaling his classmates with tales of blood and trauma.

Despite mounting concerns from the group of five students who dared to question his motives, Michael's academic brilliance shielded him from scrutiny. Yet, their suspicions only deepened as they witnessed his disturbing fixation on violence and death.

Their fears eventually found voice in the halls of authority, triggering an investigation into Michael's extracurricular activities and unsettling interests. But as the truth teetered on the precipice of revelation, the group hesitated to disclose the incidents of resuscitation and death, grappling with the inconceivable notion of Michael's involvement in such dark deeds.

Michael's excuses unveiled his true nature as a consummate liar. He asserted the necessity of a side job to support himself following his father's recent passing, a fact, and his purported need to fend for himself, a falsehood. Had the committee scrutinized his story, they would have uncovered that his mother, now holding a lucrative position as a business manager alongside her substantial widow's pension, was indeed contributing to his education expenses.

Despite their apprehensions, the committee opted to have a psychiatrist evaluate Michael's character. Yet, their apprehension over potential legal ramifications against the university prevailed over the psychiatrist's concerns. Michael had already been given free rein over patients for three years. The only repercussion he faced was the requirement to repeat a year of studies. It marked the beginning of a pattern in which Michael repeatedly evaded consequences.

In the meantime, he was ousted from his position at the ambulance service for an outburst that involved kicking a kitchen cabinet and advising a heart attack patient to seek their own means of transportation to the hospital.

Denied a Second Chance

At the tender age of 28, Michael Swango, hailed as a diligent student, attained his coveted medical degree, setting his sights on the most demanding of specialties: neurosurgery. Yet, his choice raised more than a few eyebrows, given his less-than-stellar performance in the pathology lab, where precision was paramount. Undeterred, Swango packed his bags and ventured two states away to Ohio in pursuit of his surgical dreams.

However, his tenure in the realm of neurosurgery proved short-lived, marred by his brusque demeanor towards patients and a disturbing fascination with the darkest chapters of human history, the Nazis and the Holocaust. Confronted about his unsettling beliefs, Swango responded with a bizarre display, collapsing to the ground and embarking on a series of push-ups, as if seeking absolution through physical exertion.

As word of Swango's oddities reached his supervisor, inquiries were made to the Medical School, revealing a troubling detail: Swango had repeated a year of schooling, a fact that cast doubt on his suitability for the demanding field of neurosurgery.

Denied a chance second, Swango's tenure took a sinister turn, marked by a string of inexplicable deaths within a mere 26 days. Miraculously, three patients were revived from the brink of death, but one astute head nurse, alarmed by the sudden spike in mortality, took matters into her own hands. Preserving two syringes found near the last victim, she sought validation for her suspicions.

However, her quest for truth collided with the hospital's impending windfall, a generous donation earmarked for a new oncology clinic. Eager to avoid scandal, her concerns were brushed aside, her warnings dismissed as fanciful notions. With her access to patient records denied and any mention of involving police swiftly quashed, Swango's shadowy actions persisted, shrouded in a veil of secrecy and suspicion.

Yet, the head nurse remained wary of Swango, her unease so profound that she hesitated to walk her dog alone at night, fearing potential repercussions. Despite her preservation of the syringes found near the last victim, no further action was taken, and eventually, she disposed of them, her concerns left unaddressed.

Meanwhile, a young nurse trainee, who dared to openly criticize Swango and kept sandwiches with her name in the department fridge, suffered inexplicable bouts of nausea and headaches, symptoms that inexplicably vanished whenever Swango was absent. In June 1984, nearly a year after his arrival, it was decided that Swango's pursuit of specialization must cease. Yet, fearing a potential lawsuit from Swango himself, no obstacles were placed in his path regarding his future career prospects.

Undeterred, Swango sought to expand practicing in the state of Ohio, marshaling unsuspecting physicians to provide references. Two offered glowing commendations, extolling Michael's medical prowess and patient rapport, while the third expressed reservations, but his concerns were never pursued. Consequently, Swango was granted permission to continue practicing medicine in another state.

Ricine

Just before Swango embarked on his neurosurgical specialization a year earlier, he began dating a divorced nurse with three children in Illinois. Despite his relocation to Ohio for his hospital specialization, maintaining intensive contact. However, when circumstances forced him to leave his Ohio post, he returned to Illinois to be closer to his girlfriend. Once again, he resumed his role as an ambulance nurse, this time for a different company, as he was not yet registered in Illinois. But even here, among his new colleagues, he stood out like a sore thumb. Especially his demeanor a curious blend of detachment and fascination with calamity. His delight seemed to peak amidst chaos, relishing the urgency of life-or-death situations as the ambulance blazed through the streets towards the hospital.

During downtime at the station, he paced restlessly, eagerly awaiting the next call. Eagerly volunteering for extra shifts and spending his precious days off monitoring police radio calls, often arriving at accident scenes before the ambulance. If missing an accident, he would interrogate his colleagues for detailed accounts of the extent of the injuries, a rather peculiar interest for someone trained to save lives.

Yet, behind this facade of medical duty lurked a sinister motive. In late September of 1984, Swango orchestrated a series of toxic treats for his unsuspecting coworkers. From poisoned Kentucky Fried Chicken to tainted donuts and spiked soft drinks, each offering left a trail of illness in its wake, as his colleagues succumbed to severe headaches and bouts of vomiting, one after the other.

But as suspicion mounted, Swango's carefully crafted facade began to crumble. His overt inquiries into the health status of the victims only served to draw attention to his involvement. Despite the whispers of doubt among the staff, their concerns were swiftly dismissed by their superiors, shielding Swango from the scrutiny he rightfully deserved.

Then, Swango's colleagues devised a plan, and he walked right into their trap. In secret, they kept some of the tea he had refused to drink, discovering ant poison in his bag. When arsenic was found in the tea, Swango was promptly arrested. A search of his residence unveiled a scene of chaos, a laboratory stocked with various poisons, including the deadly seeds of the tropical castor oil plant containing ricin, alongside suspicious chemical compounds, poison recipes, a firearm, and library books detailing medical serial killers. Two days after his arrest, Swango was released on bail, thanks to his family's efforts, with his mother staunchly believing in his innocence.

Undeterred, Swango wasted no time. Despite facing official charges for seven attempted poisonings, he had already secured his medical license for Ohio and applied for a position as a physician in the Emergency Department of a hospital in the northern part of the state. His job interview went smoothly, naturally omitting any mention of the ongoing investigation. The hiring committee was impressed by his credentials, ambulance experience, and passion for emergency medicine. Presenting his glowing references, Swango easily convinced them, donned his white coat, and began his new job.

However, just five weeks into his tenure, news of his charges reached the staff of the emergency department, leading to his immediate termination.

Terror Strikes

The news of the charges for seven counts of attempted poisoning reaches the hospital where Swango prematurely ended his neurosurgery specialization, sending shockwaves through the staff. Could there be merit to the ignored suspicions of the head nurse? How could legal and public relations damage be mitigated?

Fear brewed as the hospital administration, sensing impending crisis, convened with legal counsel. Simultaneously, the wary eyes of law enforcement turned towards the institution.

Even so, their inquiries were met with a fortress of resistance. Swango's personal files, the very key to unlocking the truth, were shielded behind walls of privacy concerns.

Undeterred, detectives pressed on, driven by a relentless pursuit of justice. Their pursuit uncovered a chilling parallel: Swango's unsettling past, shadowed by suspicions of nefarious deeds. The head nurse's bold step in alerting authorities further sustained their resolve.

Patient by patient, survivors emerged from the shadows, their testimonies painting a harrowing portrait. Each injection administered by Swango seemed to cast a sinister spell, leaving victims gasping for breath, as if ensnared by unseen tendrils of paralysis. Meanwhile, the silent records of the departed whispered tales of agony, of bodies ravaged by inexplicable bleedings or marred by the telltale signs of ricin's deadly touch. Nonetheless

Swango's dark fascination with the lethal toxic remained buried within the pages of his academic past.

When the internal investigation report of the Ohio hospital is finally published, its revelations will be nothing short of chilling. The conclusion will starkly state that, in the tragic cases of the four deaths and the three resuscitated patients, the possibility that someone deliberately administered a harmful substance cannot be ruled out. While the report acknowledges that hospital staff did not actively cover up the matter, it highlights a disturbing oversight: far more attention should have been given to the patients who insisted they had received a 'Swango shot'.

The report delves deeper, pointing out that nurses' statements about seeing Swango tampering with IV tubes were dismissed. This negligence is compounded by the troubling fact that the now-destroyed syringes were never properly investigated. Consequently, the report strongly advises full cooperation with the nearly completed criminal investigation.

Still, despite numerous interrogations, the investigative team has frustratingly little to show for their efforts. The most they have is the recurring detail that Swango was seen with the patients shortly before their conditions worsened. But as the detectives well know, such contact, in the context of a professional relationship, is virtually worthless as evidence. It's a maddening dead end, where suspicions run high but proof remains elusive. The prospect of charging someone for these heinous crimes grows dim, shadowed by the sobering reality that without irrefutable evidence, justice may never be served.

Ant Plague

The trial against Swango about his series of toxic treats for his coworkers begins in Illinois. The court only has access to circumstantial evidence, because no one saw that the suspect put poison in the food of the ambulance nurses. The stored tea had been in a wardrobe for two days. But a seller at the garden store points out Swango as the one who bought ant poison; he was easily recognizable because he had been wearing his uniform.

In a moment of apparent candor, he revealed a tale of battling a relentless swarm of ants within the confines of his apartment, a seemingly innocuous detail that would soon become a damning piece of evidence.

As the defense called upon an expert witness from the realm of pest control to corroborate Swango's account, the courtroom held its breath, awaiting the revelation that would tip the scales of justice. Yet, as the expert took the stand, a damning revelation came to light: the presence of red ants, native only to the southern reaches of America, defied logic within the confines of Swango's northern abode. With each probing question from the prosecutor, the facade of innocence began to crumble, painting a damning portrait of deception.

In a stunning turn of events, Swango was ultimately found guilty on five of the seven charges, his fate sealed as he was led away in handcuffs, leaving behind a trail of shattered trust and betrayed innocence.

However, Swango's release from prison doesn't mark the end of the saga. His girlfriend remains steadfast, but his mother, burdened by the ordeal, refuses to finance any further legal battles, succumbing, some say, to a heart shattered by her son's actions. Consequently, Swango sees his hard-earned medical licenses in Ohio and Illinois stripped away.

While Swango is in prison, his girlfriend remains unwavering in her support. Upon his release in August 1987, after serving two years for good behavior, they move to Virginia together. Determined to resume his medical career, Swango applies for a license to practice in the state. However, his past catches up with him, and his application is denied due to his criminal record.

Undaunted, he secures a job as a counselor at an employment agency. Where his colleagues soon find him peculiar, disturbed by his habit of flipping through scrapbooks filled with photos of gruesomely mutilated bodies during work hours. The office's unease turns to alarm when three of his coworkers fall ill with symptoms of poisoning, with one even requiring hospitalization.

Suspicion quickly falls on Swango. One of the victims files charges against him, but the investigation stalls, never advancing beyond initial interrogations. Sensing the walls closing in, Swango attempts to escape his past once more by submitting a request to change his name, hoping to slip away from the growing cloud of suspicion surrounding him.

Charm

In the spring of 1989, a peculiar figure emerged in the corridors of a coal company in Virginia. Draped in an aura of charm, Michael Swango, now a free man after a pause behind bars, applied for a position as a technical laboratory assistant. The company's director, enthralled by Swango's charismatic demeanor, eagerly extended an offer of employment.

Swango and his girlfriend tie the knot, but marital bliss proves elusive. Swango's interest in his wife wanes steadily; he demands a separate room in their home, spends hours glued to his computer, and impregnates a woman he meets at a nightclub. Meanwhile, at the coal company, a coworker and the director fall violently ill, suffering from debilitating headaches and relentless vomiting.

After two tumultuous years of marriage, Swango's wife welcomed their divorce with open arms, relieved to be rid of his deceitful grasp, especially upon discovering her depleted bank account.

Undeterred by the fallout of his failed marriage, Swango continued his enigmatic journey as an ambulance attendant in Virginia. Unbeknownst to his employers, his past remained shrouded in mystery, his actions between 1985 and 1987 left unquestioned.

Amidst the sweltering heat of the summer of 1991, Swango's path crossed with that of a new paramour, a younger, divorced nurse with fiery red curls. Not fleeing upon glimpsing the state of his apartment could only be described as miraculous. With Swango residing alone in the bathroom, accompanied only by a television and a mattress.

In early 1992, Swango secured a position at a hospital in the state of South Dakota. Together with his new girlfriend, settling into a quaint detached house after the moving truck had departed. However, their idyllic haven was soon disrupted by the resurfacing of Swango's dark past. After six months, news of his conviction reached the hospital's administration, presenting Swango with an ultimatum: resign voluntarily or face dismissal. Opting for personal resignation not only suited Swango's agenda but also spared the hospital the looming threat of lawsuits.

The abrupt termination blindsided his fiancée, particularly unsettling as she now bore the burden of their livelihood. As headlines blared across newspapers detailing the suspension of a doctor with a concealed history, the engaged couple found themselves besieged within the confines of their home, hounded by relentless media hawks stationed outside their doorstep. In a defiant display of bravado, Swango emerged from their sanctuary, chest puffed out, proclaiming, 'I am an excellent physician'. Seeking refuge, they retreated to a hotel for three weeks, yet his fiancée's condition continued to deteriorate.

Shortly after Christmas that year, she stumbled upon a prescription for poison among her partner's papers. Financially drained and emotionally shattered, she returned to Virginia, her heart heavy with despair. Tragically, shooting herself to death after a telephone conversation with Swango. Though the contents of this final conversation remained shrouded in mystery, traces of poison were discovered woven into her luscious red locks during the autopsy, a silent testament to the toxic grip of Swango's influence.

Continuing Odyssey

The 'excellent physician' showed little remorse for his fiancée's tragic demise. He remained preoccupied with scouring job listings, undeterred by the weight of personal loss. As fate would have it, in the waning days of June 1993, a military hospital on Long Island beckoned with a vacancy, a mere hour's drive from the bustling metropolis of New York. Dr. Swango, with his checkered past, approached the hiring committee with a brazen admission of his conviction, cloaked in the guise of a wrongful judgment.

Astonishingly, his confession didn't repel the committee; rather, it kindled a sense of admiration for his purported candor, unwittingly ushering him into their fold.

But the tranquil facade of Long Island's medical haven belied a sinister truth. Within four short months, the hospital corridors whispered of two untimely deaths, casting a foreboding shadow over Dr. Swango's tenure.

The details of these final fatalities, shrouded in uncertainty and dread, painted a grim tableau of suspicion and intrigue. In one case, the echoes of tragedy reverberated years later when a post-mortem examination unveiled a sinister presence, a lethal dose of nicotine concealed within the victim's mortal frame.

Meanwhile, the widow of the second victim bore witness to a harrowing scene, the sight of Dr. Swango administering a fatal injection into her husband's very veins. After which he abruptly fell unconscious and paralyzed, succumbing two weeks later. Upon learning of, as he calls himself in this hospital: Doctor Kirk's suspension due to a criminal past as reported in the newspaper, the widow sounded the alarm, only to be met with indifference from the hospital.

As the long arm of justice, embodied by the *Federal Bureau of Investigation* (FBI), closed in on Dr. Swango's trail, the stage was set for a dramatic showdown. Yet, in a twist of fate worthy of a suspense thriller, the elusive doctor vanished into the night, staying with a friend in the southern state of Georgia and seemed to be employed as a laboratory technician at the water board. That doesn't seem like a good idea and the FBI discovers his whereabouts and arranges for his dismissal by telephone.

Undeterred by the specter of impending scrutiny, Dr. Swango's odyssey continued unabated, weaving a web of deception and despair across state lines and international borders, leaving a trail of shattered lives and unanswered questions in his wake. By the end of 1994, he had fled to Zimbabwe, welcomed with open arms due to the acute shortage of medical professionals in that part of the world.

Zimbabwe

As the 41-year-old physician stepped off the plane onto Zimbabwean soil, a gesture of gratitude took him to his knees, his lips pressing against the earth in an almost reverent kiss. He had bestowed upon himself the age of 27, a peculiar detail among many others that would soon come to light in the intricate tapestry of his deceptive life.

His initial month at the remote Mnene mission hospital unveiled unsettling truths about his expertise, or lack thereof, in obstetrics and general surgery. It wasn't long before the hospital director, recognizing the gaps in his colleague's skill set, deemed it necessary to transfer him to the bustling Bulawayo hospital, a significant distance away.

In Bulawayo, his frenetic pace and abrasive demeanor raised eyebrows among his colleagues. His tireless work ethic, though admirable, his abrasive language sends shockwaves through the hospital corridors, earning him more than a few sideways glances. Yet, despite his abrasive demeanor, his insatiable appetite for work earns him a glowing testimonial upon his return to Mnene in May 1995, a development that fails to elicit his approval.

Although, his reunion with the Sisters of Mercy is anything but harmonious, marred by complaints of his brusque mannerisms and condescending treatment of non-white staff members. As whispers of his nocturnal wanderings through the hospital wards begin to circulate, unease permeates the once-tranquil confines of Mnene.

As tensions simmered, a series of unsettling incidents rocked again the tranquil atmosphere of Mnene: six deaths and two troubling incidents that rattled the medical community to its core. Faced with mounting concerns, the Swedish medical director reluctantly called upon the authorities to investigate.

A meticulous search of Swango's residence uncovered a trove of medical instruments and countless vials of medication, concealed amidst a labyrinth of soiled doctor's coats. The once-welcomed physician was summarily dismissed.

In the intricate web of Michael Swango's deceit, each chapter seems more chilling than the last. By November, he's wormed his way into the corridors of a hospital in Bulawayo, Zimbabwe, offering his services without asking for a dime. The administration, eager to fill its ranks, blissfully overlooks the ominous warnings whispered by the medical director from Mnene. One wonders why a seasoned doctor, capable of commanding hefty paychecks worldwide, would volunteer his skills gratis. But, amid Swango's seemingly magnanimous gesture, tragedy lurks. Three patients meet their end under his care, their deaths shrouded in suspicion.

Despite the chaos swirling around him, Swango finds time for dalliance, entangling himself with a divorced woman and her four children, spinning a web of lies to keep his facade intact.

But by July of the following year, Swango's carefully constructed world begins to unravel. His departure from the Bulawayo hospital, prompted by the leak of investigations at Mnene, marks the beginning of a dark spiral. In the quiet confines of his girlfriend's home, a strange malady grips the household. Her family and even their landlady fall victim, their bodies succumbing to a mysterious toxin later identified as arsenic.

Swango then looks for work in neighboring African countries. Giving a lecture at a school about what it means to be a doctor. The children loving him clapping their hands as he says goodbye. By late August, he crosses the border into Zambia and South Africa, where he allegedly secures employment in two more hospitals.

Even so, his international journey comes to an abrupt halt in June 1997 when his new employer in Saudi Arabia mandates his travel through the United States. At Chicago airport, authorities finally apprehend him.

Amidst mounting suspicions of up to sixty murders, the prospect of proving them all becomes increasingly doubtful. Initially convicted of forgery, a crime punishable by just three and a half years in prison, Swango faces the possibility of walking free in July 2000 at the age of 45.

Nonetheless, just before his release, he faces charges for nine murders spanning fifteen years, to which he brazenly confesses. Yet, he is only convicted for three and one attempted murder. Nevertheless, he receives three consecutive life sentences, shielding him from extradition to Zimbabwe.

23.

Favorite general practitioner

Harold Fred Shipman, England, 1974

Camouflage of Evil

In the vast landscape of crime, few horrors cut as deeply as those perpetrated under the guise of trust and compassion. Across the globe, tales of serial killers haunting the corridors of healthcare remain rare but chilling. Yet, nestled in the quaint town of Preston in Northern England, a sinister saga unfolded, shattering illusions and leaving scars on the souls of an entire nation.

The enigmatic figure at the center of this tale is Dr. Harold Shipman, a name that sends shivers down the spines of those who dare to remember. Born into the humble embrace of a working-class family, Harold's journey was marked by an unsettling arrogance that set him apart from his peers. But it was his descent into darkness that would etch his name into the annals of infamy.

As accusations of heinous acts cast their shadow over him, disbelief gripped the loyal patients who had entrusted their lives to their beloved 'Fred'. How could their caring physician, draped in the cloak of respectability, be implicated in such horrors? The truth, as always, proved more insidious than the mind could fathom.

However, it always remains a mystery why he chose the least obvious means, morphine, to murder his victims. As a medical professional, he must have known that this substance could be detected even after a long time. Shipman, who, like the perpetrator from the previous chapter, is after his conviction known by his surname, operated under the extremely sophisticated camouflage of what I call the Mother Teresa Syndrome. Hiding behind a mask of servitude, he applied pressure bandages to his own bleeding heart.

Tragedy

Born into the quaint English town of Nottingham on January 14, 1946, little Harold entered the world amidst the embrace of a respectable working-class family. His father, a diligent truck driver, provided for their modest needs while his mother tended to the hearth, pouring love onto her brood of three. Among them, Harold held a special place, earning the title of his mother's favorite.

From his earliest days, Harold exhibited a pedantic nature, donning bow ties and parading about with an air of knowingness that set him apart from his peers. His academic diligence was notable, though tinged with an arrogance that kept others at arm's length. Despite his struggles to keep pace with the curriculum, he found solace and distinction on the sports field, particularly excelling in the rough and tumble of rugby matches, where his fervor left spectators breathless.

Yet, tragedy loomed on the horizon, casting a shadow over Harold's final year of high school. His mother, battling cancer, became reliant on morphine injections administered by her physician. When she succumbed to her illness, Harold's reaction was shockingly detached. He fled into the night, jogging aimlessly through the rain as if to outrun the weight of his grief. From that moment onward, the specter of loss would haunt his every step.

At the tender age of seventeen, Harold embarked on his journey to university in Leeds, setting his sights on a career in medicine. It was there, during his daily bus ride to university, that he encountered Primrose, a young woman toiling away in a local haberdashery shop. Their whirlwind romance soon led to an unexpected pregnancy, much to the chagrin of Primrose's skeptical mother. Undeterred, Harold and Primrose forged ahead, exchanging vows and shouldering the weight of parenthood at a tender age.

Deadly Addiction

As Harold delved deeper into his medical studies, the pressures of family life weighing heavily upon him. And it was at the age of twenty-two, while toiling away as a junior doctor, Harold fell victim to the insidious allure of morphine, succumbing to its addictive embrace.

Thus began a downward spiral into the depths of addiction, as Harold's once-promising career and idyllic family life unraveled before his very eyes. Little did anyone suspect that behind the facade of a dedicated physician lurked a cold and calculating killer, his addiction to morphine paving the path to unspeakable horrors.

At the tender age of twenty-three, Harold Shipman proudly dons the title of doctor, embarking on a journey that would plunge him into the darkest depths of human depravity. For three more years, he labors within the confines of his training hospital, a period during which his second child, a son, is born, driven by a desire to serve as a glimmer of hope in the community, he joins in 1974 the Todmorden group practice in Yorkshire. His arrival breathes new life into the faltering practice, his enthusiasm contagious as he introduces cutting-edge medical advancements. Yet, Shipman is ill-suited for the collaborative nature of a group practice. He shuns teamwork, dismissing the involvement of practice nurses with a casual wave of his hand.

As whispers of discontent swirl among his colleagues, Shipman's demeanor darkens, his once bright spirit clouded by the shadows of inner turmoil. He claims to wrestle with depression, citing conflicts with colleagues as the source of his distress. However, those who share his professional space have no recollection of such strife, casting doubt upon Shipman's narrative.

It is within the walls of this seemingly ordinary practice that Shipman's descent into madness begins. With each passing day, the line between healer and harbinger of death blurs, until, in a moment of calculated malevolence, he commits his first murder. One life extinguished, followed by five more in the ensuing year, a sinister pattern emerging in the wake of Shipman's deadly deeds.

It was 1975 when whispers of concern first echoed through the halls, as Shipman's frequent bouts of illness raised eyebrows among the staff. But it was the astute observation of the receptionist that uncovered the true extent of Shipman's deception, a liberal prescribing of morphine that bordered on the suspicious.

Unveiled, Shipman's addiction to the potent drug could no longer be hidden. With a calculated cunning, he manipulated pharmacists, exaggerating dosages to secure excess morphine for his own clandestine use, even resorting to outdated ampules in his desperate quest to feed his cravings.

In a desperate bid to maintain his facade, Shipman turned to his colleagues, imploring them to keep his addiction and theft of narcotics under wraps. Yet, their sense of duty prevailed, and they refused to be complicit in his deceit. The consequences were swift and damning, a conviction for prescription forgery, theft of narcotics, and a partial professional ban, accompanied by mandatory rehabilitation.

But even in the face of such damning evidence, Shipman's grip on his profession remained unbroken. Despite knowing about his addiction, the Medical Board failed to expel him from their ranks. Todmorden's youth see their dealer leave with regret since he illegally supplied them with amphetamine through the back door.

Professional Ban

Forced into rehabilitation, Dr. Harold Shipman's fall from grace seemed inevitable. Meanwhile, his wife Primrose sought refuge with her mother, desperate to shield her children from the storm brewing within their family's walls. Despite her mother's pleas, Primrose could not resist her husband's attraction, and after he was released from the clinic after two years, she cut all ties with her own family to be at his side again.

With his medical license revoked, Shipman's prospects looked bleak. But necessity breeds innovation, and in 1977, he found himself as an occupational physician in the Yorkshire coal mines. However, this role is short-lived. Apparently, there is a lack of oversight regarding his professional restrictions and in a twist of fate, Shipman stumbled upon an opportunity, a position at a group practice in Hyde, a suburb of Manchester. It was here that he faced a crucial moment, a job interview with six colleagues who held the power to grant him a second chance. With unwavering honesty, Shipman laid bare his troubled past, revealing his history of addiction in a bid for redemption. Little did his colleagues know, they were opening the door to darkness.

While his peers managed patient rolls of no more than 2500, Dr. Harold Shipman's practice burgeoned beyond 3000 in no time.

Suspicious Familiarity

His success wasn't merely due to medical prowess; Shipman possessed a charm that endeared him to all. He didn't just treat ailments; he listened intently, extending consultations well beyond the typical twenty minutes. Known to all as 'Fred', he fostered a familiarity that erased barriers. In return, he addressed everyone by their first names, a gesture of camaraderie that endeared him further.

Rejecting any semblance of pretension known by doctors, Shipman chose to sit beside patients, engaging them with playful banter and jokes, even flirting with older female patients, all the while earning their unwavering loyalty. Despite his occasional brusqueness when his advice wasn't heeded without question, patients were captivated by his charisma, willing to follow his directives unquestioningly. Take what the doctor advices and stop complaining, is his motto. Meanwhile prescribing twice as many medications as an average GP.

Shipman's popularity soared, particularly due to his willingness to make house calls, a practice that, in hindsight, takes on a sinister turn. To his patients, his request to remember his practice in their wills seemed innocuous, just another quirk of their beloved doctor. But behind this facade of amiability lay a dark truth, a web of deception that would soon ensnare all who crossed his path.

Dr. Shipman was hailed as a hero, a tireless crusader in the fight for life, his zeal for emergencies unmatched. Skipping meals to attend to patients, he exemplifies dedication. While his colleagues delegated responsibilities during off-hours, Shipman insisted on being on call at all times, even redirecting patient calls to his home after hours and on weekends. His commitment extended beyond the medical realm, with active involvement in community affairs, serving on the school board and volunteering to train ambulance personnel.

But beneath this facade of dedication lurked a darker truth. Shipman's inability to maintain professional boundaries became evident, his colleagues observing with growing concern. His fervor could swiftly turn to fury, particularly when met with resistance. His superiority complex often led to clashes, with nurses and secretaries bearing the brunt of his ire. A trivial dispute led to an eighteen-month silence with the practice manager, highlighting his inability to navigate interpersonal relationships.

Yet, amidst the chaos, Shipman remained an enigma. His private life shrouded in mystery, visitors seldom crossed the threshold of his home. Even in his rare moments of leisure, Shipman eschewed hired help, opting to repair his roof himself.

Private Practice

Within the confines of the group practice in Hyde, two extraordinary phenomena remained shrouded in secrecy. Firstly, the unsettlingly high mortality rate among Dr. Shipman's patients went unnoticed, alongside the resurgence of his addiction to morphine. Shipman, ever resourceful, devised cunning schemes to fuel his dependency, resorting to deception by fabricating cancer diagnoses to justify prescribing excessive amounts of morphine, each dose disappearing into his own grasp. He also scavenged ampules from the deceased, a sinister tactic employed by those with nefarious intentions in the healthcare realm.

As Shipman approached his forty-sixth year, the atmosphere in the group practice grew increasingly fraught. Then, in a shocking turn of events, he brazenly established a private practice named 'The Surgery,' a mere stone's throw away down the same street. With audacious disregard for his colleagues, he absconded with all his patients and financial assets from the group practice, leaving his former colleagues burdened with debt and resentment. Moreover, he callously refused to contribute to their collective tax obligations, a further betrayal that underscored the depths of his duplicity.

Even within the walls of his private practice, Dr. Shipman retained the adoration of his patients, their unwavering loyalty. Amidst the chaos of a disorganized patient administration, Shipman found solace in his newfound freedom, with only Primrose managing the front desk.

Even so, behind this facade of devotion, upsetting reality unfolded. Patients were dying with alarming frequency, their deaths shrouded in mystery. Despite the staggering toll of lives lost over decades, few dared to question the beloved 'Fred'.

Rumors

It wasn't until the last few years that whispers of unease began to surface, two souls brave enough to heed their instincts and reach out to authorities.

Among them, a taxi driver, his heart heavy with suspicion as he noticed a pattern among his elderly passengers, each one a patient of Shipman's, each one suddenly missing. His concerns dismissed by others, he eventually mustered the courage to approach the authorities in 1996, his plea for investigation met with little more than a passing glance.

In early 1997, a conversation between a funeral director and his daughter, both intimately familiar with Shipman's clientele, sparked further unease. They couldn't shake the unsettling image of the deceased, found fully clothed in their chairs, one sleeve often rolled up, a detail that raised more questions than answers.

The household members of the funeral director, all patients of Shipman, sternly forbade him from meddling further. But with a quiet determination, the man brushed aside their warnings, marching straight to the general practitioner's office to lay bare his concerns. Shipman, with a cool attitude, placated the undertaker, assuring him that all was well.

As the year progressed, two astute GPs began to piece together a troubling puzzle. One couldn't shake the feeling of Shipman's unnerving presence at the bedside of the dying, while the other noticed a curious pattern in Shipman's mandatory requests for additional checks before cremations. Yet, it was the meticulousness of Shipman's own examinations during second opinions for colleagues that raised the most eyebrows. His joking remark to the undertaker about leaving no stone unturned only added to the hostile atmosphere.

In the early months of 1998, the two doctors made a bold move, taking their suspicions to the authorities. However, a superficial investigation led the police to attribute the elevated death rate to Shipman's elderly clientele. Even the home care organization couldn't ignore the alarming number of fatalities, yet remained inert.

Only much later did the truth begin to surface, revealing that Shipman's patients themselves harbored concerns about the disproportionate number of elderly women meeting their end prematurely, their absence felt keenly at the bridge table. But fear stifled their voices, leaving their suspicions to fester in silence.

Pigs

In the sweltering heat of June 1998, the truth about Doctor Shipman, aged 52, came to light as he administered a fatal dose of morphine to his latest victim. By the time the lifeless body of the octogenarian woman was discovered, meticulously arranged on the sofa, Shipman had already tampered with her medical records on his computer, trying to paint a picture of long-standing morphine addiction. Little did he know, every keystroke was etched into the digital tapestry, leaving an indelible trace.

The daughter of the deceased, herself a seasoned attorney, couldn't shake her doubts about the explanation given by the family doctor. Especially unsettling was the revelation that her mother's will had been clandestinely altered just before her passing, leaving behind a fortune for Shipman. And the forgery was so clumsy, it practically screamed foul play. Fueled by suspicion, the lawyer took matters into her own hands, summoning the authorities to launch a thorough investigation.

The police, spurred into action by mounting evidence and past suspicions, descended upon Shipman's domain. Two undercover officers paid him a visit, blissfully unaware of the tangled web they were about to untangle. Meanwhile, a separate team scoured his residence for clues. Shipman, ever the picture of composure in his practice, brazenly denied any wrongdoing, insisting only on speaking to the chief police officer. The policemen couldn't shake the memory of Shipman's courteous manner as he bid them adieu, holding the door open with a disarming smile.

When news of suspicion flooded the airwaves the following day, the strain became palpable for the doctor, particularly in the presence of a patient. Although, that very afternoon, he effortlessly faced a reporter, his performance betraying no hint of concern.

Meanwhile, the police, sensing the urgency, desperately sought ways to halt Shipman's practice. Despite the swirling accusations, even after his visage graced the front pages, he continued his consultations. His patients, blissfully unaware of the tempest brewing around their cherished 'Fred', remained steadfast, convinced he had merely granted euthanasia to a few tormented souls. They even cast a shadow of resentment towards law enforcement, who dared to disturb their beloved 'Fred's' tranquility. Even following Shipman's arrest, flowers continued to flood in, and the waiting room bulletin board remained a testament to their unwavering loyalty.

Shipman's employees, once blindly devoted, transitioned into vital allies for the investigative team.

As detectives combed through Shipman's residence, they were met with a scene straight out of a nightmare. The pervasive stench of neglect mingled with the peculiar sight of pig ornaments strewn throughout the cluttered rooms. It seemed as though neither broom nor duster had graced the premises in months. Not a clean cup in the cupboard. The investigative team later left speculating that Primrose, Shipman's wife, may have unconsciously sensed her husband's nefarious deeds and simply given up trying to keep things in order.

Amongst the disarray, incriminating evidence lay hidden, jewelry and trinkets belonging to Shipman's victims, and in the garage, a trove of patient records and a stockpile of morphine awaited discovery. With evidence in hand, Shipman was promptly apprehended, but the mysteries surrounding his actions were far from resolved.

Weight of Truth

As investigators dug deeper into Shipman's murky past, it became increasingly evident that the shadows enveloping him stretched far beyond a mere forgery. In the interrogation room, the doctor adopted an air of indifference, brazenly defying the gravity of the situation. He refused to offer his name for recording, his responses veering into the realm of absurdity. When he grew weary, he turned his face to the wall, a silent protest against the relentless questioning. After six grueling hours, he casually inquired about going home, oblivious to the fact that his freedom was slipping away forever.

Subsequent interrogations unraveled his facade. Tears flowed as the charges of three murders echoed in the stark room. Shipman's appearance shifted, his head swaying gently as if rocked by an unseen tempest. His words, once confident, dissolved into incoherence, his body collapsing under the weight of his guilt. Yet, amidst the chaos, he vehemently denied any wrongdoing.

Even in the confines of his cell, Shipman's behavior remained enigmatic. Fearful of poisoning, he shunned sustenance, relying solely on the apples tenderly brought by Primrose. Letters penned in desperation reached out to those he believed still harbored faith in him, former colleagues, as well as, incredibly enough, relatives of his victims. In each missive, he adamantly proclaimed innocence, painting himself as the victim of a grievous error. In verse, he bared his soul to his wife, lamenting the abyss of loneliness engulfing him.

Primrose and her children remained steadfast in their support, never wavering their silence in the face of public scrutiny. Yet behind closed doors, Primrose tirelessly assisted investigators, determined to uncover the truth. Whether she harbored any involvement in two murders would forever linger in the shadows, for she was never brought to trial.

Meanwhile, the investigative team burned the midnight oil, with fifty-nine dedicated detectives tirelessly pursuing leads. A hotline was established, inviting individuals to report any suspicions, and soon, the roster of potential victims swelled. As the full extent of the tragedy emerged, disbelief transformed into dejection among the residents of Hyde. At the train station ticket counter, in the cozy corners of local pubs, and amidst the aisles of bustling demeanor to have a personal connection to someone who had fallen under his care. How could such a pillar of the community, someone they trusted implicitly, be responsible for so much heartbreak?

With each revelation, the community recoiled in horror. Autopsy after autopsy confirmed what had once been unthinkable: Shipman's patients had not succumbed to natural causes as reported; instead, they had been victims of lethal doses of morphine. As the body count climbed, the magnitude of the devastation became painfully clear.

Echoes of Deceit

Slowly but surely, the harsh reality begins to penetrate the minds of the grieving, unlocking doors to memories long suppressed. In Todmorden, a relative of one victim suddenly recalls the coldhearted encounter with

Shipman at the door, forcefully pushing past her with the claim that he was merely there to determine the cause of death, her father, though ailing, hadn't drawn his last breath. With a brusque entrance into the bedroom, Shipman made a swift exit, leaving behind a haunting void. It was mere minutes later that the woman discovered her father's lifeless form.

In another haunting tale, a newborn's life is tragically cut short shortly after a home birth. The mother, receiving an excessive dose of morphine by Shipman prior to the delivery, watches helplessly as her baby struggles to breathe. Despite the dire situation, Shipman adamantly refuses to transfer the infant to the hospital, fearing his deeds would be uncovered. Aware of Shipman's hand in their daughter's loss of life, the grief-stricken parents choose silence, swayed in part by Shipman's feigned distress.

And in a somber twist, a 67-year-old diabetic woman is discovered lifeless in her chair by her husband after Shipman's visit. Frantic, the husband reaches out to Shipman, only to be met with an unexpected lack of concern. Shipman's dismissive presence, without even a cursory examination of the deceased, leaves the husband bewildered. With a disconcerting assurance, Shipman dissuades the husband from involving the authorities, promising to handle the situation himself.

In the cases of other victims, it emerges that the doctor consistently marked on forms that he had conducted external examinations, a claim disputed by family members. They noticed how the GP avoided coming into close contact with the deceased, never laying a hand on the body again.

Yet, amidst the horror he inflicted, Shipman remained strangely composed. Accounts surfaced of him eagerly orchestrating proceedings, even theatrically summoning an ambulance, a mere facade later exposed by meticulous scrutiny of phone records.

During one episode, Shipman administers a lethal dose of morphine to a patient home alone, heartlessly leaving the building, casually taking her sewing machine under his arm. Through a twisted fate, he meets the patient's unsuspecting brother, who is unaware of her fate. Shipman callously informing him of her death and brazenly claiming that she had promised the sewing machine to Primrose. and that he already takes it with him.

Harold Shipman's behavior harbors a confounding contradiction. While projecting an aura of superiority to colleagues and investigators, he seeks to dissolve barriers in his office, striving to be not just a physician, but a confidant and companion to his patients.

Thrice

In the heart of Shipman's practice, a anomaly unfolds: five patients breathe their last within its confines, a rarity in the realm of family medicine. Shipman's later account paints a grim picture: he claims to have spent a quarter of an hour valiantly attempting to revive one of them, yet strangely, he neglects to enlist the help of his receptionist or dial for an ambulance. Instead, he seamlessly transitions to attending to the next patient, leaving the deceased to rest in the adjacent consultation room.

But the saga takes an even darker turn when Shipman embarks on a grim spree, claiming three lives in a single day. The first victim, feeling unwell, seeks solace in a call to the doctor, only to find him at her doorstep, uninvited. A mere half-hour later, she breathes her last.

Without pause, Shipman flits back to his practice before venturing out again, this time to the home of the second victim. As the afternoon wanes, Shipman makes a third visit, this time witnessing the passing of the third patient in his care. It's a tableau of tragedy, leaving the families of these victims shaken and profoundly affected by the supposed compassion of their doctor.

For Shipman, these macabre acts seem to unfold most frequently in the hush of the afternoon, between 2:00 and 4:00 PM, a sinister routine where sixty percent of his victims succumb within a half-hour after they unsuspectingly let him in.

The unnerving swiftness with which Shipman's patients met their ending following his visits defies the norms of medical practice, especially considering none were in the terminal stages of illness. Nonetheless, Shipman's methodical approach to obfuscating the time of death reveals a precise calculation. Post-injection he would crank up the heat, ensuring the bodies remained warm upon discovery, a deliberate ploy to sow confusion. Moreover, his aversion to autopsies and insistence on cremation only deepen the veil of secrecy shrouding his actions.

As the list of victims unfolds, a troubling pattern emerges: one that suggests Shipman had a sinister preference for targeting those who dared to oppose him. One patient adamant about keeping her husband out of a nursing home is silenced. Similarly, a vulnerable patient who dares to question the doctor's treatment of his son meets his end on a somber Christmas Eve. Despite the lethal dosage of morphine, Shipman's victims are ushered into the great beyond without a trace of fear or pain, enveloped in the deceptive warmth of their trusted confidant. Moments before Ruth, Lilly, and Elisabeth take their final breaths, Shipman soothes them with false promises of preventative measures, like antibiotics or vitamins.

Adding Up

In the quiet town of Todmorden, Shipman's deadly tally begins, claiming the lives of six patients during his brief tenure of one year. Yet, it's in the bustling group practice of Hyde where his alarming deeds truly flourish, with at least 66 souls meeting their untimely end over fifteen years. Then, in the solitude of his solo practice, Shipman's lethality reaches a horrifying crescendo, as an additional 143 patients fall victim to his lethal touch in just six short years. A simple observation reveals a chilling trend: a slight lull after Todmorden followed by a disturbing surge, with the rate of murders escalating from 0.5 to nearly 2 per month.

The surge in killings just before Shipman's unmasking could perhaps be explained by the phenomenon where serial killers, sometimes utterly losing their grip (if they hadn't already), become increasingly sloppy, almost as if begging to be caught. It's almost as if it's a cry for help. As Whittle & Ritchie aptly put it in their book *Prescription for Murder* (2001): Shipman had to draw attention to his crimes, for what would be the point of being the greatest murderer of all time if no one knew? The clumsy attempt at forging his final victim's will serves as yet another eerie piece of evidence supporting this theory.

As the courtroom falls silent, the presiding judge delivers a sobering verdict: beyond the confirmed 215 victims, including a disproportionate number of women, there likely lies a hidden toll of another 45 lives lost. Yet, even with such staggering numbers, the true extent of Shipman's atrocities remains elusive, forever shrouded in the shadows of uncertainty.

Control

Throughout the trial of Doctor Shipman, his conduct demands scrutiny. There's an unsettling effort on his part to maintain a veneer of control. Each day, as he enters the courtroom, he exchanges a casual wink and nod with Primrose and the children in the gallery, almost as if he's off for a leisurely outing. Clutching a stack of papers under his arm, a gesture more befitting of his attorney, he takes his seat. While the court proceedings unfold, he appears diligent, scribbling notes as if to capture every detail. Yet, it's later revealed that his scribbles amount to little more than idle doodles and tic-tac-toe games to while away the hours.

When Shipman himself takes the stand, he adopts the air of a learned professor, delivering his testimony with a sense of authority. Throughout the trial, he feigns difficulty in hearing, repeatedly asking the judge to repeat questions, an obvious tactic to buy time. Only once does he allow a glimpse of vulnerability, breaking down in tears as he confesses to 74 heinous acts and admits to tampering with patient records. His manipulation of records, done even before the commission of his crimes or the discovery of his victims, weighs heavily against him. However, this revelation does little to alter the course of his fate, a verdict of fifteen consecutive life sentences for a litany of charges including multiple murders, forgery, and theft. Anyhow, hearing his final sentence, Shipman remains stoic, his attitude unchanged, leaving his attorney visibly shaken.

Even during his incarceration, Shipman's need to assert control is evident. Despite his conviction, he persists in his role as a doctor, conducting consultations for fellow inmates and even prison staff. In a final act of defiance, after three and a half years behind bars, Shipman manages to exert the ultimate control over his fate, taking his own life despite the heightened scrutiny.

Perfect Facade

Shipman wore his mask with such finesse that it ensnared everyone around him. Long before his exposure, he orchestrated a cunning move, having his handwriting scrutinized by a graphologist under the pretense of seeking insights into a friend's character. The results were as disturbing as they were predictable: the author of the text was portrayed as an intelligent, dangerous, and dominant figure, adept at bending rules to his advantage.

As revealed by psychologists and psychiatrists during his trial, Shipman harbored a latent, untreatable personality disorder, characterized by rigid, obsessive traits. Driven by a profound sense of inadequacy, he hid behind the guise of the altruistic GP. But beneath the veneer of kindness lurked a cold, distant figure, his disdain for others so palpable that it poisoned every interaction. Humiliating others became his only outlet, a testament to his inner contempt. Shipman himself remained tight-lipped about his true motivations.

At least one of Shipman's motives is somewhat comprehensible to the layperson. He murders some of his victims out of base greed, long side ridding himself of troublesome individuals.

Closing words

This book is primarily written for a general audience, delving into 23 international cases to uncover the facts and shed light on the motives of the perpetrators. The described crimes hold particular relevance for professionals in the broad fields of medical and paramedical care. One critical takeaway from this book is the urgent need to take whistleblowers seriously, this change is crucial for ensuring greater patient safety when medical personnel are no longer beyond suspicion.

To gather the data, I conducted thorough research and co-authored a pivotal study with Beatrice Yorker titled *Serial Murder by Healthcare Professionals*, published in the American *Journal of Forensic Science* in 2006. My investigative journey took me to court trials, where I had access to essential court files. Additionally, my sources were supplemented with (semi) scientific non-fiction and comprehensive internet research.

In terms of privacy, except for Dutch perpetrators, all convicted individuals were mentioned with their full names, as these were obtained from public sources such as the internet, to allow readers to further inform themselves. If information on the perpetrators was not publicly available, the same discretion was applied as with the Dutch cases. To minimize imitation behavior, the most commonly used lethal means were described in veiled terms.

This manuscript was originally set to be published in 2010 by a Dutch publishing house. However, after a Dutch nurse previously sentenced to life in prison for the murder of several patients was acquitted, the publishing house withdrew its contract. Regrettably, the number of murders by medical personnel continued. Among the cases included are some of the most chilling examples:

- 2005, Niels Hogel, Germany, convicted for 85 murders, possibly 200 more
- 2010, Joan Vila, Spain, convicted for 11 murders
- 2010, Aino Nykopp-Koski, Finland, convicted for 5 murders, attempted 5 more
- 2011, Roger Kingsley Dean, Australia, convicted for 11 murders and causing several patients grievous bodily harm
- 2015, Victorino Chua, England, convicted for 2 murders and poisoning 22 patients
- 2016, Elizabeth Wettlaufer, Canada, convicted for 8 murders, 4 attempted murders and 2 aggravated assaults
- 2020, Satoshi Uematsu, Japan, convicted for 19 murders and 26 injured
- 2021, Reta Mays, USA, convicted for 7 murders and one attempted murder.
- 2023, Lucy Letbe, England, convicted for 7 murders, attempted murder 6

Writing a non-fiction book is never a solitary endeavor. Several individuals contributed behind the scenes to this final product. For years, I have relied on Dr. Wim Best, a forensic toxicologist and senior Inspector for Healthcare in the Netherlands. Additionally, Robert Forrest, emeritus professor of forensic toxicology at the University of Sheffield, England, provided me with invaluable information. I also consulted Professor Karl Heinz Beine, a psychiatrist, psychotherapist, and medical director of St. Marien-Hospital in Hamm, Germany, for further insights.

My relationship with Lecta de Noord, an andragogist and author of children's books, is of an entirely different nature but equally important. While enjoying homemade cake or a glass of wine at the garden table, Lecta meticulously scrutinized the manuscript. Thank you, Lecta, for standing by me for the fifth time in the publication of one of my books.

Above all, it is at home where my partner Theo Pronk creates the space for me to sit behind the laptop. I couldn't wish for a more willing listener and critical commentator on my texts. This demonstrates that with a little goodwill, private life and work can harmoniously coexist.

Bibliography

Beine, K.H., 'Homicides of patiënts in hospitals and nursing homes: a comparative analysis of Case series', in: *International Journal of Law and Psychiatry* 26 (p. 373-386), San Francisco, 2003

–, *Sehen, Hören, Schweigen, Patiëntentötungen und aktive Sterbehilfe*, Freiburg, Lambertus, 1998

–, 'Falsches Mitleid – Tötliche Konzequenzen, Uber Krankentötungen in Kliniken und Heimen', *Frankfurter Rundschau*, Frankfurt, 2002

–, Krankentötungen in Kliniken und Heimen, Aufdecken und Verhindern, Freiburg, Lambertus, 2010

Cauffiel, L., *Forever and Five days*, Kensington Publishing Corp., New York, 1992

Clarkson, W., Evil beyond Belief, John Blake Publishing Ltd, Londen, 2005

Elkind, P., *The Death Shift, The True Story of Nurse Genene Jones and the Texas Baby Murders*, Viking Press, New York, 1989

Enzlin, M., *Alle schijn tegen*, Bohn Stafleu Van Lochum, Houten, 2003

Field, J., Caring to Death: *Discursive Analysis of Nurses who Murder Patients*, University of Adelaide, 2007

Forrest, A.R.W., 'Investigation and Prosecution of Health Care Workers who systematically Harm their Patients', Unpublished PhD thesis by the University of Wales, 1992

Furio, J., *Letters from Prison. Voices from Women*, Algora Publishing, New York, 2001

Gibiec, Ch., *Tatort Krankenhaus. Der Fall Michaela Roeder*, Dietz Nachf, GmbH, Bonn, 1990

Haan, W. de, *Het voordeel van de twijfel*; 'Engel des Doods', radio documentary, Humanistische omroep, 1996

–, 'Tragedie in eenzaamheid', Humanistische omroep 1996

Halpern, L., 'Implications of the Clothier Report', NCBI, *PubMed, National Library of Medicine*, 2002

Hare, R.D., *Gewetenloos; de wereld van de psychopaat*, Elmar, Rijswijk, 2003

Hickey, E.E., *Serial Mass Murderers and their Victims*, Wadsworth Publishing Company, Belmont, 1991

Hoek, P.H. van der, Netwerk, *Moord en mededogen*, KRO-tv documentary, 6 november 1996

Jongsma, W., *De zaak Frans H. De rechtszaak van de eeuw*, Uitgeverij Het Land van Valkenburg, Valkenburg, 1976

Lampe, P., *Het Moeder Teresasyndroom. Het Persoonlijk Motief in de Hulpverlening*, Nellissen, Soest, 2002

–, *Engelen des Doods. Lucia de B. en Andere Seriemoordenaars in de Gezondheidszorg*, Karakter, Uithoorn, 2007

–, *Seriemoordenaars in de Gezondheidszorg*, 2014

Linedecker, C.L. en Z.T. Martin, *Death Angel, A Serial Killer Nurse's Twisted Trail of Murder*, Kensington Publishing Corp., New York, 2005

Mair, G. *Angel of Death, The Shocking Story of Charles Cullen, the Serial Killer Nurse and the System That Failed To Stop Him*, Chamberlain Bros., New York, 2004.

Malèvre, C., Mes aveaux, Fixot, Parijs, 1999

Manners, T., *Deadlier than the Male, Stories of Female Serial Killers*, Macmillan Publishers Limited, Hampshire, 1997

Moir, A., Jessel, D., *Geboren misdadigers. Fascinerende speurtocht naar de biologische oorsprong van gewelddadigheid en criminaliteit*, Kosmos-Z&K, Utrecht, 1995

Peters, C., Harold Shipman. Mind Set on Murder. Andre Deutsch Ltd, Londen, 2006

Phelps, M.W. *Perfect Poison, A Female Serial Killer's Deadly Medicine*, Pinnacle Books, Kensington Publishing Corp, New York, 2003

Ramsland, K., 'Angels of death; the nurses, Criminal minds and methods, Motives', *Crime library*, 2007

–, *Inside the Minds of Healthcare Serial Killers. Why They Kill*, Praeger, Westport Connecticut, 2007

www.robertorotondo.de, Veröffentlichungen vortrag 'Hinschauen oder wegsehen', *Der Fall Irene B.*, date unknown

Schmidbauer, W., *Die hilflosen Helfer, Uber die seelische Problematik der helfende Berufe*, Rowohlt Verlag, Reinbek bei Hamburg, 1977

–, *Wenn Helfer Fehler machen, Liebe, Mißbrauch und Narzißmus*, Rowohlt Verlag, Reinbek bei Hamburg, 1997

Smet, T. de, *Soeur Mourir*, Borgerhoff & Lamberigts, Belgium, 2023

Stewart, J.B., *Blind Eye, The Terrifying Story of a Doctor Who Got Away With Murder*, Simon & Schuster Inc., New York, 1999

Document court case Rudi Paul Z., *Az,: 30 KS 1/5 (46 / 75 v)*, Landgericht Wuppertal, August 2, 1976

Document court case Martha U., Rechtbank Groningen, December 07, 1995

Document court case Martha U., Rechtbank Groningen, April 18, 1996

Document appeal Martha U., Rechtbank Leeuwarden, October 8, 1996

Vaknin, S. en L. Rangelovska, *Malignant Self Love: Narcissism Revisited*, Narcissus Publications, Praag, 2005

Vermassen, J., *Moordenaars en hun motieven*, Meulenhof/Manteau, Amsterdam, 2004

Whalen, W. en B. Martin, *Defending Donald Harvey, The Case of the Most Notorious Angel-of-Death Serial Killer,*Emmis Books, Cincinnati, 2005

Whittle, B. en J. Ritchie, *Prescription for Murder, The True Story of Dr. Harold Shipman*, Warner books, London, G.B. 2001

Yorker, Crofts, B.A., 'Nurses Accused of Murder', in: *American Journal of Nursing*, vol. 1, issue 3 (p. 35-46), New York, October 1988

–, 'Hospital Epidemics of Factitious Disorder by Proxy', *The Spectrum of Factitious Disorder*, American Psychiatric Press, New York, p. 157-175, 1996

—, "Liability Associated with Factitious Disorders," *Journal of Nursing Law*, vol. 5, no. 4, pp. 7–22, New York, 1998

—, and A.R.W. Forrest, K.W. Kizer, P. Lampe, J.M. Lannan, and D.A. Russell, "Serial Murder by Healthcare Professionals," *Journal of Forensic Science*, vol. 51, no. 6, pp. 1362–1371, West Conshohocken, November 2006

Previous publications by Paula Lampe

Gedeelde kinderen. Co-ouderschap als keuze
(Ambo, 1998, 2nd edition 2003)

Het Moeder Teresasyndroom. Het persoonlijke motief in de hulpverlening
(Nelissen, 2002, 2nd edition 2003)

Hulpverleners in een multiculturele samenleving. Verhalen en interviews
(Nelissen, 2004)

Engelen des doods. Lucia de B. en andere seriemoordenaars in de gezondheidszorg
(Karakter Uitgevers, 2007)

Eenzaamheid begrepen. Over armoede en rijkdom van het zelf
(Nelissen, January 2009)

Seriemoordenaars in de gezondheidszorg
(Independently published, 2014)

www.ingramcontent.com/pod-product-compliance
Lightning Source LLC
Chambersburg PA
CBHW052308220526
45472CB00001B/30